MW01141316

This Adventure Called Life

Healing From Breast Cancer Naturally

Peny Goodson-Kjome

SunShine Press Publications, Inc.

SunShine Press Publications, Inc.
PO Box 333
Hygiene, CO 80533

Cover design by Bob Schram of Bookends
Chapter illustrations by Ann Franco-Ferreira
of Great Arts Originals
Author photo courtesy of Paul Jacques
Cover photo courtesy of NASA

Publisher's Cataloging-in-Publication Data

Goodson-Kjome, Peny.
    This adventure called life : healing from breast
cancer naturally / Peny Goodson-Kjome.
        p. cm.
    Includes bibliography, index, and appendix.
    ISBN 0-9615743-8-0
    1. Breast-Cancer-Patients-United States-Biography.
2. Breast-Cancer-Popular works. 3. Breast-Cancer-
Treatment. 4. Breast-Cancer-Psychological aspects.
5. Self-care. 6. Alternative medicine.
7. Naturopathy. I. Title.
RC280.B8.G663   1995   95-68183
616.99'449-dc20

Printed in the United States of America

2 3 4 5

Printed on recycled acid-free paper using soy-based ink

Dedication

To a universe of freedom with responsibility, peace with harmony and the wisdom of health and love.

Acknowledgments

To my husband, Norman Thor Kjome; editor, Hettie Jones; chapter illustrator, Ann Franco-Ferreira; cover designer, Bob Schram; publisher, Jack Hofer. Without you my book would not have been born.

And to those who also gave me their loving support. My children and granddaughter, Jamie, Jim and Paige Adams, Joel Myron May, Peter Kjome, Kristin Kjome and Jonathon Fischer, Kari Kjome and Catherine Kjome, my parents, Myron and Marjorie Goodson, my brother and family, Ralph, Pat, Matthew and Amy Goodson, my friends, teachers, analysts, healers, and clients.

I love you all. Thank you.

Contents

Foreword

To many, the diagnosis of cancer is the greatest shock ever experienced, "Oh my God, I'm going to die!" If the initial shock ever wears off, it turns to resignation and acceptance. Peny, however, through her inner being, took the moment and transformed her diagnosis to, "Oh my God, I want to live!"

I appreciate the opportunity to write the foreword to Peny's book, for it has moved me to reexamine my own attitudes toward cancer and the nature of life-threatening challenges. Both of my parents died of cancer. In fact, it has been the cause of death in every close relative. I was still a child during the years of my mother's illness, repeated mastectomies, chemotherapy and radiation. I can clearly remember her misery, most of it from the effects of her treatment and the inability to be present for her four children and her husband. To this day, almost twenty years later, I remember her crying with our family about the time she could not spend with us because she was so sick. Despite the treatments that broke us financially and emotionally, she died. She died away from us. It is this I remember. With hindsight, I wish those years of illness could have had some aspect of "quality of life" for her, myself and the rest of her family.

Peny once told me, during one of our many discussions, that her body had been trying to tell her something for years, but she chose to ignore it. Her cancer was the wake-up call to pay attention to herself. To really pay attention to her needs and to what was important.

This book is part of that process. Peny has a strong desire to share her path with others confronting a life-threatening illness, not to say her choices are the best or only way, but to encourage them to wake up and pay attention. Now! Today!

Naturopathic philosophy holds that the Creator gives us wonderful bodies with a capacity to keep in balance. Without this capability, we would have died out as a species long ago. When out of balance, the body informs us by creating symptoms which bring awareness. If we choose to ignore these messages or forcibly remove the symptoms without a healing process, our bodies will find another way to bring the imbalance to our awareness, usually through a deeper illness. For some, the end stage pathology is cancer, the ultimate imbalance.

The dominant medical approach to cancer is surgery, chemotherapy and radiation. These are useful in the mechanical treatment of the tumor and some associative processes, but they in no way affect the cause. To be truly healed, one must address the cause—perhaps toxic exposure (environmental and/or medicinal), nutritional imbalances, lifestyle or emotions. The process of healing is the unfolding of understanding toward ourself, our nature and life.

Peny takes her wound and wears it like a magic crystal that speaks to and guides her. It awakens and makes her aware when she is acting out-of-balance and subsides when she is in accordance with herself and life. Peny's vision is colored by this crystal as it brings each day into sharp focus. It is a gift of clarity and purpose.

Peny has taught me much about being human, confronting my darkness and places of fear. Her power of being, at times, is intimidating. After a few meetings with her, I remember thinking, "I'm sure glad she likes me." When she first came to my office, I knew right from the beginning she wanted a helper in her process, a support for her needs. At no time was she going to give up her personal power or turn her life over to me, the physician. Peny showed me my true role as a physician—a partner in the healing process. I could not heal her and she knew that. The power to heal resided within herself. I was to act as her coach, share knowledge, monitor progress, cry together, touch and most important, be a willing participant on her path of healing.

When confronting a life-threatening challenge, at some level we must enter the darkness, not knowing whether we have made the right choices. It is critical that we make these choices from the center of our being, so that the chosen therapies resonate with us. It is not so important what we choose for treatment, but that this choice is compatible with our inner being.

We will all die. How we live is how we die. The quality of our existence determines the quality of our death. If we are in alignment with ourselves, our ability to make the right choice is much clearer.

As we enter the closing of this century, cancer continues to be a leading cause of death despite the billions of dollars spent in finding a cure. No cure will ever be found looking outside the body. Disease created from within must be healed from within. This is the lesson Peny has learned.

In health,
Michael Lang, N.D.
Kalispell, Montana

Introduction

Peny has found her body and her healer within. Her story is a voice to so many others who are listening for a new sound that will sing the truth to them. Sing loudly, Peny! We are thankful for your gift of courage.

—Chris Griscom, *Founder and Director of The Light Institute*
Galito, New Mexico/St. Severin, France

I am not a physician, psychiatrist, or priest. Everything described in this book is my own personal experience.

In September of 1991, my doctor told me I had breast cancer. Two weeks before, a good friend of mine had died. I believe he did not die exclusively from the effects of cancer, but that the medical treatment he received played a big part. I did not want that to happen to me. I decided, instead of traditional treatment, that I would use alternative methods of healing, loving my body to health instead of doing battle with it and dying slowly hooked to a morphine drip as had my friend.

Some people in our culture believe healing is learning to die gracefully. For me, healing meant becoming healthy. I was not afraid to die. Living, whole and healthy, was my desire.

I became enraged over how our culture treats cancer. Standard procedure is to do surgery, chemotherapy and/or radiation. Women's breasts and men's testicles are often removed. Then they are told, "Be happy, you're alive." Not for me, thanks.

I am a Jungian psychotherapist. Several years ago I studied Jungian Psychology with Clarissa Pinkola Estes. When I read her book, *Women Who Run With The Wolves* (Ballantine Books, 1992), Chapter 12, "Marking Territory: The Boundaries of Rage and Forgiveness," it made sense to me. In her book, she suggests that to be healthy it's important to transform your rage into something positive. I have taken my rage about cancer treatment and transformed it into this book.

This is *my* story about breast cancer. I am *not* recommending any specific traditional or alternative treatment. I want everyone to know there are choices—not to do it my way, but to do what is right for you and to live, in health, each day.

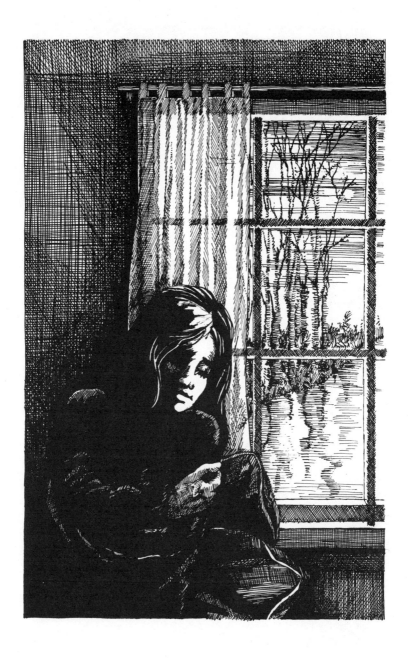

CHAPTER ONE

Cancer

Discovery, diagnosis and my decision to live

On September 2, 1991, while standing in my living room talking on the phone and casually doing a breast exam, I discovered a lump in my left breast.

Nothing felt casual to me now. I could hardly breathe. Adrenaline surged through my body. I hung up the phone and felt again. Yes, there *was* a lump in my left breast. Bile welled up into my stomach and the back of my throat. My bowels loosened and I barely made it to the bathroom. I sat there, trying to think.

I'd better call my doctor. I made my way back to the phone and called. "I've just found a lump in my breast. Does the doctor have any time today?" I held my breath. *Please*, I prayed.

The nurse was back immediately. "We've had a cancellation. You can come in at 1:00 p.m."

I sat down, trying to decide if I should call Norman, my husband, or wait until he came home for lunch.

I had married for the fourth time, after years of analysis and learning about myself. I'd been divorced, widowed and divorced. It took five years of courting by a very special man before I felt safe enough to marry again.

I decided I'd wait until lunch. After all, it was only a lump. Women got those all the time. Why did I feel so afraid?

At lunch, my husband repeated the same thing. "You'll be okay, sweetheart," and gave me a hug.

When I arrived at the doctor's office, the nurse said it had been a while since I'd been in. Two years! I couldn't believe it. I always get a Pap smear every year. "Not last year," she said. She's right, I thought to myself, I was too busy planning my daughter's wedding to take time to go to the doctor.

The doctor did the exam and told me to dress and then to come into his office. Standard procedure. That's what he always did. I dressed and went in to see him. He was abrupt with me, which was very unusual. He'd been my doctor for years and always took time with me. "I want you to go down the hall to the surgeon and have that lump biopsied. It looks bad to me and I don't think you should waste any time."

I was trying unsuccessfully to take a deep breath. My hands felt slick as I gripped them together. I looked at him and heard myself saying, "I'll go to Denver. I want to go to a specialist."

"Don't take too long about it," he said, "and let me know what he says."

I stood up, walked unsteadily to my car, and drove to my husband's physics laboratory. He turned, took one look at my face and put his arms around me. I clung to him, not able to speak or cry, just hanging on. After a bit, he stood back and asked me to tell him what the doctor had found. I said we had to go to Denver as soon as I could get an appointment.

"Go home and make the appointment. I'll be home soon," he said.

All the way home I prayed. The energy force I pray to, I call The Creator. That force, in my family, is called God. As I grew older and began to see God as all-encompassing, I became more comfortable with the term The Creator. In my heart The Creator included Mother, Daughter and Soul with Father, Son and Holy Spirit. This seemed more balanced because it connected me to the earth as well as to the heavens. The Creator is very personal and sacred to me, as I trust it is for everyone. When I pray, I hear a voice, inside me, that I always have trusted was The Creator, speaking with me.

I was thinking, as I pulled up to my house, that it was interesting how things happened. A month ago

I'd been visiting with a friend whose mother had died of breast cancer. She told me she was going to the best oncologist in the Rocky Mountain area. I called her as soon as I got home and she gave me his name and telephone number.

The woman who made the appointment for me seemed warm and understanding. She scheduled an appointment for me a few days later. On the day of my appointment Norman and I drove to Denver. The doctor's office was near our favorite Greek restaurant, so we went there for lunch before going over for my biopsy.

We arrived early. The women in reception were very helpful and I began to relax. They took me to an examining room and I was told to remove my shirt and bra. The nurse asked me several questions about my medical history. The doctor came in just as she finished.

"We're going to do a needle biopsy," he said. "You should get your results in just a few days." He went on to say how he used to ranch but couldn't make enough money. Now, however, he was making plenty of money. He told me to lie down on the table and said this wouldn't take long.

Searing pain flashed through my breast as he began his probe. He was having trouble getting what he wanted so he repeated this procedure several times. By that time I was near tears and trembling all over. "What's the matter, are you nervous?" he asked. I couldn't reply. I had seen people go into shock. That's how I felt, distant from myself and cold. The doctor finished, told me to get dressed, spoke with me as I did so and then told me to come to his office. Shivering, I had gotten back into my bra and shirt. When I walked into the reception area, Norman saw me and immediately came to my side. The nurse directed us to the doctor's office. We sat together grasping hands. I was shaking so hard I could hardly sit on my chair. My husband acted as though he would have liked to pick me up and run from the office.

The doctor said that the biopsy wouldn't be back for a few days but he felt sure I had cancer. He said he figured I knew it too. I nodded, yes. Then he gave me a book that he said would explain surgery, chemotherapy and radiation treatment. He went on to say that I could wait two weeks for surgery but he strongly recommended against waiting.

The pathology report showed—*Fine needle aspiration cytology: Positive for malignant cells. The malignant cells noted in the smears as well as the cell block are consistent with origin from infiltrating duct carcinoma of breast origin.*

When I realized that he was booking me for surgery, in just over a week, without any more discussion and no other choices, I wanted to leap over the desk separating us and beat on him with my fists. I wanted to kill him. At the very least I wanted to scream at him, "Whose life do you think this is, you son-of-a-bitch!

This is my body! Don't sit there so smugly pronouncing my death sentence. How dare you drop me into this place of terror."

All these feelings and thoughts buffeted my body, increasing my agitation. Norman, feeling my energy, abruptly stood up, gently pulled me to my feet and helped me to leave the doctor's office.

We went to our car and drove to my daughter's home, which wasn't far from the doctor's office, where we all clung to one another and cried. Jim, my new son-in-law, was blown away. His Mom had died of cancer when he was twelve years old and he couldn't believe his new Mom had just been diagnosed with it. I told everyone I needed to go, so we all hugged and Norman took me home.

After we arrived, I went into the bathroom and stood washing my hands looking into the mirror. There I was, dead. The pupils of my eyes were steel grey, not black. I remembered that this was how my second husband's eyes were after he had been killed in a motorcycle accident.

I stood there, transfixed. As I stared at my reflection, the voice I recognize as The Creator said to me, "That's right, Peny, you can go right now or you can stay. I know you've been unhappy with the world, all the violence, pollution and injustice. If you want to go, you can. If you want to stay, however, you may. Violence, pollution and injustice will still be here and you won't get any special treatment, but if you want to stay, do it. Which will it be?" With no hesitation I said, "I want to LIVE." Black replaced the steel gray of my pupils and I knew my spirit had returned to my body. My task, now, was to learn how to become healthy.

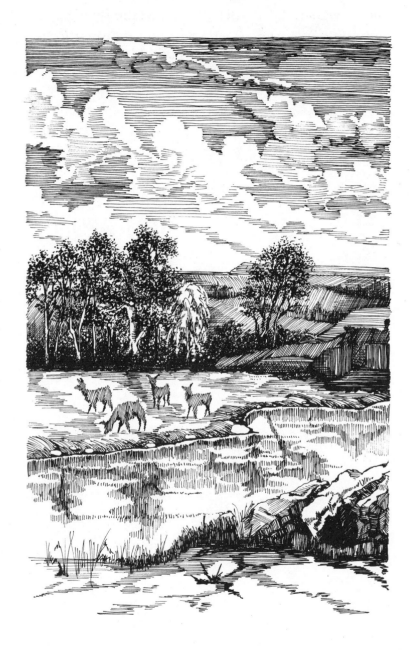

CHAPTER TWO

Decisions

Getting clear about
what path to take

not only wanted to live, I also wanted responsibility for my own life. I certainly didn't want to turn myself over to doctors who didn't seem to realize that this was my body, and that I might know something about how I felt and what was going on with me.

On the day of my biopsy, I realized I wanted to talk with my college roommate. She'd been living with cancer for many years and I wanted her advice. I called from my daughter's home and said I needed to see her. "I just had a biopsy and I need to talk with you about cancer."

I heard her take a deep breath. "Do you want to come tomorrow?" she said.

Linda lives about four hours from me, so I figured I could easily get there by early afternoon. "Tomorrow will be great, thanks. I'll be there by two."

"It will be easiest if you call when you get to town," she said. "Then I'll guide you to my house."

"Thanks, Linda, I'll see you tomorrow."

Later Linda told me that after she had hung up the phone she'd turned to her husband and said, "Why does everyone I care about get cancer?"

I'm sure everyone Linda cares for doesn't, but that's how she felt. My belief is that she's here for those of us who need her because of her personal experiences.

The spring before my diagnosis Linda had come to my home for a visit. When we were freshmen in college, we'd been best friends. During the next thirty years, we'd only seen one another occasionally. Last spring, while we'd visited, she'd shared with me that she'd had cancer twice and that both her mother and mother-in-law had also been diagnosed with cancer. She had held their hands while they'd died.

When I called her after my biopsy, I trusted that she would talk to me honestly. She, unlike the doctors, wasn't in a position to make money from any choices I made.

The day of my trip dawned partly cloudy but with no rain. As I drove, staying with the flow of traffic on the interstate, I remembered a client of mine who had told me about visualization. She said that many years ago she'd been diagnosed with cancer and had been completely cured visualizing a tiny cell, similar to the Pac-Man video game character, eating her cancer cells.

I knew several therapists who successfully used visualization with their clients and I had also read Shakti Gawain's book, *Creative Visualization* (Bantam Books, 1983). As I was thinking about how I might use this information to help with my own healing, I passed a truck hauling part of a huge dump truck, the kind used in coal mines. Its tires were bigger than my car. There, I thought, I'll visualize trucks hauling away cancerous cells and dumping them into my waste system where they'll be expelled. Since snake, to me, symbolically represents healing and knowledge, I decided snakes would bite off the mutated cells and spit them into the truck which would dump them. I spent the rest of my trip visualizing busy snakes and miniaturized powerful trucks running throughout my body, working for my healing.

When I arrived, I pulled into a gas station to call Linda so she could come get me.

She arrived soon after my call. I walked over to her as she was getting out of the car. We hugged. I followed her home and we sat down for a serious talk.

"Peny," she said, "there are a couple of things I want to say right away because I see you're very distressed. The first thing I want you to know is that you have time to decide what choices you want to make."

"But the doctor has already scheduled me for surgery," I said. "He told me I shouldn't wait over a week, two at the most."

Her look was grim. "That really makes me angry," she said. "I've been working with and learning about cancer for sixteen years. When you find a lump yourself, like you did, you've probably had the cancer three to five years. You have plenty of time to think carefully about what you want to do. After all, you're looking at a decision that will have a powerful impact on the rest of your life."

Tears spilled down my face as I realized how scared I'd been of having surgery in a week. "What else can you tell me?" I asked.

"I had a complete mastectomy a few years ago when my doctor saw the shadow of a tumor in one of my breasts," she said.

I gasped, "Wasn't that pretty severe?"

Linda looked at me steadily. "Maybe," she said, "but you need to remember that I sat with my mom and my mother-in-law as they died. I believe Mom died from chemotherapy and my mother-in-law from radiation treatments. I knew I had to do anything to avoid either of those experiences."

I nodded my head in agreement.

Not only had I witnessed my good friend's death, my brother's friend had died within a short time after his cancer treatment. I agreed with Linda completely. That whole process of chemotherapy and/or radiation treatment seemed in opposition to what I understood of healing.

"There's one other thing, Peny," Linda said. "You will learn to say no or you will be dead."

Clear and to the point. I liked that. Quietly I sat with her words. Intense emotion filled my chest as I realized it had taken a diagnosis of cancer before I would allow myself to say no to all those people who wanted something from me.

I felt fear loosening its grip as Linda lovingly shared more of her experiences.

"Peny," she said, "I know a couple who take an herbal compound that they are convinced cured her breast and his colon cancer. Would you like to meet them?"

A small surge of energy moved up from my stomach into my breasts. That energy felt like hope. "Yes," I said, "I'd like to meet them today."

Linda called and asked if we could come to the couple's home. They said fine.

When we arrived, Linda introduced me. Both were in their late fifties. Silver streaked their hair. Their bodies were solid, neither too thin nor too fat. Their good health was apparent in their glowing skin, sparkling eyes and energy. I hoped, one day, to look and feel that good.

The woman told me they'd been diagnosed with cancer twelve and seven years ago and had chosen to take the compound instead of doing the traditional methods of surgery and chemotherapy. She also explained the compound.

"Peny," she said, "You'll feel like hot snakes are running through your body. That will be the compound of herbs cleansing toxins from your system. Cleansing is necessary if you are to be healthy."

She was right. That's exactly how I felt later when I took the compound, flushed of toxins and brought to health. I found it very interesting that on the drive that had led to meeting these two, I had been visualizing snakes helping dump trucks cleanse my body.

Her husband showed me how much compound to take and when to take it. "If you want some," he said, "a three month supply will be $25."

I spent the night with Linda and her husband. Cancer had impacted both of them in different ways. They shared honestly with me their fears, joys and insights they'd gained because of their experiences. I left believing I had begun a path to health.

My next door neighbor owns a bookstore. She'd read a book written by Dr. Susan Love, one of the foremost breast cancer specialists in the country. I'd taken Dr. Love's phone number from the book and called her clinic on the east coast. She recommended a woman doctor in a city closer to my home. Since my biopsy had been positive, I had made an appointment for further consultation.

When I returned from Linda's, I told Norman I couldn't possibly go to another doctor. I felt so violated and betrayed by my doctor contacts that I believed one hospital stay would kill me. Not rational, I realize, but that's how I felt.

Decisions

The morning we were to go for the consultation was clear and beautiful. I took a deep breath, turned to my husband and said, "Let's tell everyone we're going to the doctor so they'll relax and let's go to the hot springs instead." The spring is a free natural mineral hot spring called the Hobo Pool.

"Whatever you need," he said. "I have to go to work first, but we can leave at noon."

For years I had been reading books about being connected to the earth and Native American spirituality, written by Sun Bear, an American Indian Medicine man. I took a book he'd written with others titled *Walk in Balance* (Prentice Hall Press, 1989), our swimming suits and my herbal compound. When we arrived, we checked into a room and began the process of deciding what I wanted to do for myself and what my husband needed as well. In a situation like this, it's often harder for the spouse than the person diagnosed. After all, if I died, I'd be gone. My husband would be the one left alone. We knew that these decisions would have to be shared.

We soaked in the hot pool, walked along the river, watched the deer graze near a golf course, made love, read and talked. While by the river, I lay down with my chest in the sand and committed my imbalance (cancer) to the earth and her healing. My husband explored the edges of the golf course and we both looked for lost golf balls. Relaxing together helped release us from the terror of my diagnosis.

I was no longer experiencing terror, but fear would return at odd times. That evening, after a walk by the river, we went to eat supper. As I looked at the menu I burst into tears. There was no hot food listed that didn't include red meat, white flour, sugar and salt. In *The Handbook of Alternatives to Chemical Medicine* by Mildred Jackson, N.D., and Terri Teague, N.D., D.C. (Lawton-Teague Publications, 1985) I'd read that fresh fruits, vegetables and grains were recommended for people with cancer. Red meat, white flour, sugar and salt should be avoided. That made sense to me, but I felt starved for something hot to eat. I settled for tomato rice soup with a beef broth base, trusting that the beef broth would be okay this one time. The next morning, after a breakfast of plain, hot oatmeal, I began to feel better and less weepy.

In *Walk In Balance*, Sun Bear speaks of an initiation often being accompanied by a very hard task. That got my attention. I remembered, even in my fear, that I had been praying, for several years, to become a healer. I had always gotten what I prayed for even though it did not always look like what I believed I had prayed for.

As I had cried and screamed my fear at the time of my diagnosis, the voice inside me that speaks from The Creator said to me, "Pen, I needed your attention. Do I have it?"

Indeed!

Decisions

I remembered I had prayed unceasingly not to have anything happen to my children, or to my husband, and also not to be in a wheelchair. I had sensed that I was due for another major life change. Three of the last four times I'd experienced major changes, I'd lost a husband. I didn't want that to happen this time. The wheelchair prayer had been added after I'd fallen down my basement stairs and cracked two of my ribs. The pain had been so intense that I lay there thinking maybe I'd just die. Then I'd realized that this would be a cruel thing to do to Norman. He would come home from work and there I'd be, all stiff at the bottom of the stairs. After that experience, I understood that at any moment I could be crippled. I hadn't learned yet that life has to do with paying attention. I hadn't been ready to accept responsibility for my own life. I was going along letting life happen to me instead of being responsible for living my life every day. The day I discovered my lump I accepted this responsibility.

It's hard for me to explain just how clearly I understood that not only my breast, but my whole body had cancer. Because this was clear to me, I began thinking about every resource available to help the whole body. Norman agreed with this choice.

When we got home, I believed I could not heal with a lie between myself and most of the people I valued. I sat down and wrote a letter to all my family and my dearest friends. I'm including the letter here because it illustrates the clarity I had gained in a short time.

My loved ones' concern for me felt very heavy and I wasn't sure I could bear the weight. My initial intense fear, my turning away from prescribed treatment, my diet of fruits, vegetables, nuts and grains plus everyone's concern combined to make me feel quite fragile. I knew that if I were going to survive to become healthy, I had to be in relationship with those people who could honestly support my choices. I'd have to stay away from everyone else, pray unceasingly and take care of my body.

On the day I had originally been scheduled for surgery, I wrote this letter:

September 25, 1991

Greetings Family,

I am writing one letter and duplicating it so I only have to do this once. If I had to do it over, I'd be tempted not to tell anyone. Cancer, in our culture, engenders a hysterical reaction and everyone's concern feels like anvils dropping onto me from all directions. The weight of everyone's fear has been horrific.

I know, in my heart, that you all love me. I love you too, and have been blessed with your loving. Many other times you had no idea what I was up to but you loved me anyway, and for that I thank you. I am blessed that my husband and children support me one hundred percent.

Decisions

About thirteen years ago, after my last divorce, I made a complete connection with what I perceive to be God.

My God is an androgynous, all encompassing entity I call The Creator. I don't speak with you all about my spirit because it feels very personal but I'm connected. I've known, in my heart, that I could withstand anything given to me and I can. I didn't wish to call in difficulty but here it is.

I have been praying unceasingly for a couple of years that I might be allowed to transform from mother/nurturer to healer. This cancer is my rite of passage toward that goal. My psyche and spirit are in great shape, my emotional is so-so, and my physical a disaster. My attention is now totally focused. I am tending to my emotional by getting clear and finally taking care of my physical. I needed a severe jolt; I got it.

Mom and Dad raised me to be honest with myself and others. My kin were pioneers and very strong. Consequence—when I know something and it's important that I be honest with my "self," I am intensely strong toward that end. Dr. Carl G. Jung was giving a lecture one day when he was asked if he believed in God. His response was, "No." Everyone was shocked and disturbed. After a short silence, he said quietly, "I know!" That's where I am with my cancer; I don't believe any particular thing, I know what I must do for myself in order to be well.

*In my private practice as a Jungian psycho-
therapist, I work as a conduit through which The
Creator passes information to my clients. They heal
and live their personal power. I can do no less for
myself.*

*My body is my temple on this planet. I must work
with it, not against it. For people who are comfortable with the traditional medical community,
standard procedure sometimes works.*

*For many of you, surgery, chemotherapy and or
radiation would be the answer. It is not mine. I
believe that my whole body has cancer, not just my
left breast. I know you want me to prove it with
medical tests. I'm telling you that by the time I
experienced all the tests necessary as well as spent
that amount of time in a hospital I believe I would
die. That's how I feel.*

*I do not wish to die so I am doing many things to
cleanse myself of toxins and to enable my whole
body to be well. I am connected to physicians in
Wisconsin and Mexico who work with cancer
healing all the time. My primary contact is with a
nutritionist, who is advising me as I change how I
eat and learn what vitamin and mineral supplements to use. I'm taking an herbal compound that
detoxes my body and pancreatic enzymes to help my
digestion.*

*I believe that everyone has cancer cells but that
when your immune system is healthy it destroys*

*those cells before they can mutate. I am doing
everything I know of to strengthen my immune
system.*

*Two years ago I began flushing my liver, after my
herbalist told me it was congested. Too much fat,
sugar and alcohol in my diet. I believe beginning to
detox my liver may have saved my life. My cancer
probably began in my liver and surfaced in my
breast so I'd pay attention. I've experienced pain
around my liver for several years but was too busy
to do anything about it. Besides, I figured all my pains
were pre-menopausal.*

*Do not imagine that I have not been terrified.
Having to look my own death in the eye is something
that cannot be easily explained. I can only say that
it makes having been a widow simple, and I thought
that was the worst. This is the ultimate and my
choice is to live as honestly as I can with what I'm
learning is necessary for my complete health and
well-being.*

*I did not go to another doctor. When I realized I
was only going for some of you, I canceled my
appointment. I must follow my heart, not your fear.*

*I have prayed to be able to stay in my body on this
planet. I have asked to be forgiven for betraying my
health through poor habits. I believe I can become
completely healthy.*

*I know most of you support my choice and those of
you who don't, do so from fear. Please try to release*

your fear. Let's live, bless every day, laugh a lot and have fun. This planet is magnificent and so are all of you. I love you all.

I do not wish to speak of cancer anytime soon. Be well, be happy. I pick up your energy so let it be loving.

I love you,
Peny/Mom

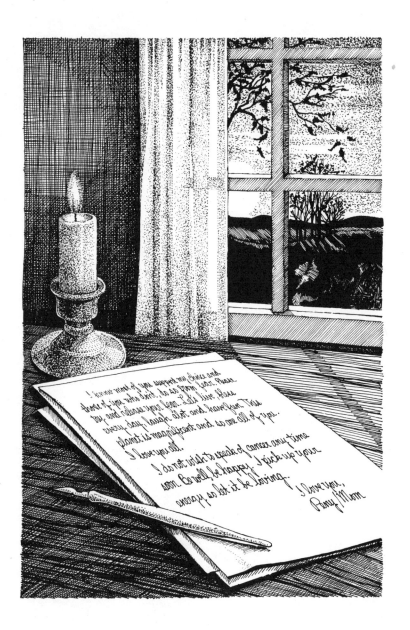

CHAPTER THREE

Changes

Choices I made and
the people who helped me

The response I received from the people in my life who are most important to me is clear in the letter my brother sent:

September 26, 1991

Hi there,

We just got your letter so I decided to see if you still read. I've been trying to call for a while and it would appear that either you've left or don't answer your phone anymore. Contacting you seems a bit difficult.

I understand your reluctance to talk to people because you don't want to be yelled at, but don't shut us all out, okay? We are also concerned and not just a little afraid.

We are, of course, kind of stranged-out over your approach to healing yourself. We're pretty traditional, you know, and this isn't what one normally finds in the doctor's office. That said, I must now say that as one who spends a lot of time promoting an individual's ability to control their own destiny through the power of the mind (mind over matter type of approach) that to not support you would be massive hypocrisy. So, consider yourself supported.

I'm really not trying to be flip, or maybe I am because I'm scared and being flip is a way to shut out the fear. But anyhow, while I may not choose your route for myself, I certainly understand your approach to healing by using your own capabilities and not those of a professional doctor type who probably doesn't know shit about you or your psyche. (I have no idea how that is spelled, my spell checker is going to have a ball with this when I'm done.)

We are all terrified that you will die and we don't want that to happen. You're one of the good people and not just because you're my sister. The world needs more of you, not less. Be patient with us and we'll endeavor to be the same with you. When you get your act grouped, or if it is already, get in touch, okay? . . .

Love,
Ralph

The rest of his letter was wonderfully funny and I laughed; long, loud and from my belly. What a terrific feeling. The loving, honest, humorous support that came to me from family, friends and clients was one of the most important reasons I had the courage to take responsibility for my life. The thirteen years I'd spent in Jungian dream analysis and trust in my herbalist were also very important factors.

I had sought the counsel of this herbalist two years before, when I had been feeling out of sorts. She did a thorough workup on me and learned that my liver was congested. One of the functions of the liver is to help with the metabolism of carbohydrates, fats and proteins. For years I had abused my body with too much fat, protein and alcohol. The result was that my liver was no longer metabolizing effectively, which my herbalist called congested. Instead of flushing toxins, I was holding them in my system. With her guidance I had begun a program for cleansing and detoxification using herbal remedies. She also gave me Bach flower remedies to help with my depression. Dr. Bach, in his book, *The Bach Flower Remedies* (Keats Publishing, Inc., 1979), said that the basis of disease is disharmony between spiritual and mental aspects of a human being. He prepared remedies, using flowers, that relieve mental distress until problems can be dealt with from within. Unfortunately, the only change I made in my diet was to give up chocolate. I believed using the herbs, flower remedies and giving up chocolate was all I had to do. This was the program I was following when I was diagnosed.

My son was outraged. How could I get cancer, he asked, when I'd been using the herbs? I told him that herbs alone couldn't keep my body healthy. Proper diet and exercise were essential for me to be well and I hadn't realized that until now.

My husband never wavered in his support of my doing exactly what I knew was right for my life. One evening, soon after my diagnosis, his brother called. Norman's brother is a medical doctor and he was concerned that I wasn't going to have surgery. He was yelling at my husband, saying, "It's standard procedure." I loved Norman's reply.

"Peny isn't standard," he said, and hung up the phone.

My task was to learn to take care of my physical body. For years I'd believed I had been. I'd say to my clients, "I practice what I preach." And I did, as far as my psyche, intellect and spirit were concerned. I had a library filled with books about health and healing, but hadn't applied what I knew to my own body. I was chubby. I'd decided not to worry about being slender because I was nearly fifty and everyone knew you put on a few pounds as you age. Besides, I loved fat food, what Norman called glop—gravy, sauces and cheese. My favorites were pepperoni pizza, cheese and onion enchiladas, chicken fried steak or fried chicken with mashed potatoes, biscuits and gravy. I also loved a soft drink that was high in sugar and caffeine. I ate so much salt that when I'd sweat my face would form a white film. And I drank some kind of alcohol almost every day. I walked once in a while and sometimes did some dance aerobics, but I did not exercise regularly. My body was going to last forever without my taking care of it.

Wrong!

After my positive biopsy I was determined to flush all toxins from my system.

My husband had a book written by Dr. Harold J. Reilly and Ruth Hagy Brod, *The Edgar Cayce Handbook for Health Through Drugless Therapy* (Jove Publications, 1975). In it, Cayce recommended enemas for cleansing your system. I already knew that hot steam baths were good for me, so I decided I would have a cleansing day, once a week, on Monday.

Using some of Dr. Reilly's ideas, I began my Mondays with three enemas:

1) 1 quart of warm water with one teaspoon of instant coffee. This coffee enema stimulates the liver. For this enema I would lie on my left side.

2) 1 quart of warm water with 1 teaspoon of salt and 1 teaspoon of baking soda. I'd kneel with my forehead on the floor.

3) 1 quart of warm water with 1 tablespoon Glyco-thymoline, a mild disinfectant. I would lie on my right side. Changing positions helped to thoroughly flush my intestines. I took enemas a minimum of once per

week for four months, giving my body a good chance to cleanse.

Next, I made up one quart of warm water mixed with the juice of one fresh lemon. I sipped the lemon water, which helped to flush my cells, as I took a twenty to thirty minute hot bath. I put one cup of baking soda and one cup of salt in the bath water. This helped my pores to open and flush themselves of toxins. I pulled my shower curtain so that I also got a steam bath. Breathing deeply, I'd cough up mucus from my lungs.

For emotional cleansing, the next step was to cry, scream, and swear, releasing all the things I was aware of that were causing me pain, anxiety or distress. I would visualize them draining away when I pulled the plug in the bathtub.

After this, I would pray, thankful for my cleansing, healing and blessings. Often, after releasing emotional baggage, I'd burst into song or compose poetry in my head.

Then I'd put on my housecoat, wrap my head in a towel, cover up with a blanket and sit quietly. As sweat poured from my body, I'd meditate and listen to answers to my prayers. After twenty to thirty minutes, I'd take a shower, wash my hair and rinse the toxins away.

During the remainder of the day, I drank juices and ate lightly, taking a break from my vitamin supplements. Sometimes I would fast, drinking only citrus juice and distilled water. I'd rest, stay as quiet as possible and unplug my phone.

Because the lump was in my breast, I decided that my glands needed particular cleansing. I stopped shaving under my arms and quit using deodorant or antiperspirant. I was pleased when I noticed my body odor was not unpleasant. I'm sure this was due to not eating red meat or dairy products, and eating very little fat, salt and sugar.

Susan Rosoff, my chiropractor, had given me a copy of *One Answer to Cancer, An Ecological Approach to the Successful Treatment of Malignancy* (The Kelly Research Foundation, 1967) by William Donald Kelly, D.D.S., M.S., in which he recommends a diet of mostly fruit, vegetables and almonds similar to that of Jackson and Teague. I bought a juicer because I knew I'd consume more vegetables if I juiced them than if I only ate steamed or raw vegetables. Drinking carrot, celery, beet and parsley juice helped to cleanse my system, supplying vitamins and minerals as it did so.

I teased my Mom that juicing was an easy way to get her vegetables. She can barely stand to put them in her mouth and much prefers potatoes and gravy. Her mother thought the only decent vegetable was creamed corn. I didn't have to look far to see why I loved fat food.

After two weeks of raw fruits, vegetables and nuts, I realized I needed some more advice about my diet. When I asked my friends to recommend a nutritionist, two of them suggested the same woman. She lived within a hundred miles so I was able to arrange a meeting right away.

We agreed to meet at my chiropractor's office. Soon after we met, the nutritionist, Barbara Frazier, and Joelle Schumacher, who practices Feldenkrais massage and is in association with my chiropractor, did an attunement with me. One stood at my head and the other at my feet. They put their hands on me and balanced my energy between them. After they had finished, in about ten minutes, Barbara said to me, "You're starving. It will be interesting to read your tombstone, which will say, 'This woman healed herself of cancer and died of starvation.'" I laughed, pleased to hear I would be working with a woman who had a sense of humor.

She said she couldn't talk with me sensibly until I'd eaten. We went to a vegetarian restaurant where she ordered for me: green salad with miso dressing, whole grain rolls, brown rice with steamed vegetables and tofu, and chamomile tea. Hot food, what a treat. While we ate, I learned that Barbara had worked for twenty years with a doctor who treats cancer patients in a clinic in Mexico. She was in contact with a doctor who would recommend the supplements I needed. I intended to heal from my inside out, and she understood that concept.

I told her I'd been detoxing, using herbs, drinking homemade vegetable juice and walking daily. "That's good," she said. "Let me tell you some other things you can do. Put one teaspoon of salt and one teaspoon of vinegar in the water when you wash your fruit and vegetables. Any chemicals that might have been used will wash away with this mixture. You also need to get a water purifier. Drinking water that isn't contaminated with chemicals is very important for your health." She gave me one of the cookbooks she had written, which not only had recipes but a shopping list for staples that were important to eating healthfully. The list of supplements, she said, would arrive within the week. The last thing she said to me was, "Peny, you and your husband need to make lots of love. It's one of the best healers there is." I was glad to hear she had common sense to complement her sense of humor.

After I had eaten healthfully for a while, I put together a plan I call "Outline for Healthy Eating" (see appendix). This is the outline I still follow. I ate often during the day, so I wouldn't feel as if I were starving. My primary foods were fresh fruit, whole grains and vegetables. I needed animal protein, so I ate poultry, fish and eggs before 2 p.m., giving my body the chance to metabolize the protein before I went to sleep. I used very little salt, sugar or fat, and I ate no dairy products, red meat, chocolate or caffeine.

Another person I believed would help me on my path to health was a friend of mine who taught yoga. Sally Benedict had studied and practiced yoga for sixteen years and I trusted her to help me learn. She also had a sense of humor, along with the good sense to let me cry when I needed to. Some mornings, as we began our deep breathing exercises, I'd begin to sob, gulping in great breaths of air as I released more toxins from my emotional body. After I'd cried until I was exhausted, we'd continue with my lesson. Gently, she'd encourage me to stretch and come into balance once again.

On the days we worked straight through with no emotional outbursts, Sally would say, "Hear those organs giggling? They're so happy you've decided to help them do their work." I was so impressed with my organs that I named them all. Sam Spleen was my favorite, reminding me of Sam Spade the detective. I thought this was appropriate since the spleen is an organ that produces lymphocytes, which track down mutating cells and destroy them, a major function of the immune system. I'd read about lymphocytes in *The Cancer Answer*, by Albert Earl Carter (A.L.M. Publishers, 1988), a book Norman had found for me in a health food store.

I also drew all of my organs so I could visualize them in their proper places, sloughing off slime as they healed. I imagined them glowing with health as they giggled and said thank you.

A friend of mine had suggested that acupuncture might be a good idea because it also works with the organs and the flow of life energy. I went to a few practitioners, looking for someone I'd feel good with.

Margaret Helenschild was not only well versed in acupuncture and Chinese medicine, she also had a restful and supportive attitude. From her I learned that the organs all support one another. In a circle graph were spleen and stomach, lungs and colon, kidneys and bladder, liver and gall bladder, small intestine and heart, temperature regulation, circulation and sex organs. Reading around the circle I noticed that the kidneys and bladder support the liver and gall bladder. No wonder my liver was still not functioning properly; for many years my bladder and kidneys had been weakened by infections. We were both pleased when I responded well to the treatments and all my organs began to strengthen.

As I learned about and experienced alternative healing methods, I was sad and angry that none of the Western doctors I'd trusted had ever suggested any of these methods to me.

My analyst and psychic helped me stay clear about the information from my unconscious. My herbalist supervised my detoxing and my use of the Bach flower remedies. My nutritionist supported a healthy diet and appropriate supplements. Yoga stretched my muscles and tickled my organs. Massage and reflexology helped move my lymph fluids and relaxed me, which helped my attitude. My chiropractor kept my structure aligned and my naturopathic and homeopathic doctor checked my whole system. What a blessing to have such a competent, knowledgeable group of people loving me and helping me to come into balance and health.

I also learned to be quiet and by myself. I would draw a Rune or a Medicine Card and then meditate about the message. Viking Runes are an ancient alphabet whose letters have names. *The Book of Runes* by Ralph Blum (St. Martin's Press, 1982) is a handbook for the use of Runes as a personal Oracle. An Oracle doesn't give instructions as to what to do next or predict the future. It points out hidden fears and motivations, and helps a person make better choices.

Medicine Cards: The Discovery of Power Through the Ways of Animals by Jamie Sams and David Carson, illustrated by Angela C. Werneke (Bear and Company, 1988) are teachings that use animal qualities to help us as we search for unity with all life.

I honor the land and animals that Runes and Medicine Cards represent.

I had been very fortunate that when I found my lump I wasn't sick. I had been diagnosed with cancer, but I felt fine. Because I didn't hurt or feel sick, I was able to make rational choices about how I wanted to become healthy. I was also blessed with a husband and family who supported me, not only emotionally but financially. Along with learning to say no, I learned to ask for help. My parents gave me money and my husband made all his resources available to me. What good was his money going to be to him if I was dead?

Because I had that kind of support, I was able to take a year's leave from my practice of psychotherapy. I spent that year completely focused on doing everything I could to help my body become healthy. I did not do all of the alternatives at once. I did each as I learned about it or as it felt right. I spent hours sitting quietly, listening to the answers to my prayers. I'd been praying for many years, probably all my life, but I had never before taken the time to listen for the answers. All my choices now are the result of my listening to the voice in my head that I believed was The Creator.

What Linda had talked about with me, and what I came to realize, was that this cancer diagnosis was my wake-up call. I had to look carefully and honestly at how I'd been living and then make changes. My clients and I often talked about how we say we want change but then continue living in the same old ways. Change means doing things differently. I don't know that I would have been able to move toward health if I hadn't changed my way of eating, exercising, the way I thought about my responsibilities and how I worked with stress and depression. A big part was learning to say no. It was scary but also very exciting to make changes and start to move toward health.

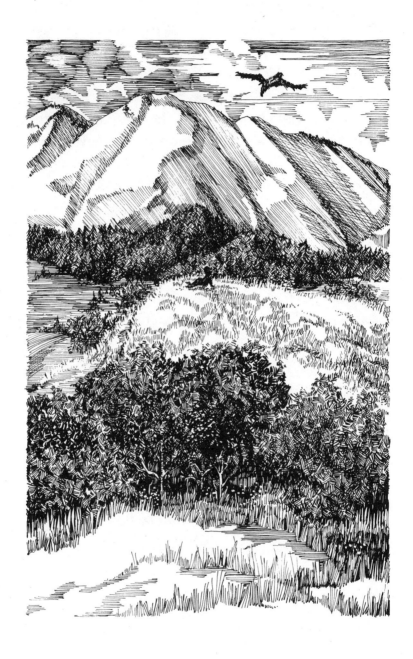

CHAPTER FOUR

Coming to Consciousness

Where I came from and who I am

My health had never been a big deal to me. I had always taken it for granted. I'd also been willful, needing to find out everything for myself, often learning the hard way.

Peny Wilberta Goodson May Boice Kayser Kjome. That was me. Peny with one *n*. My maternal grandmother's maiden name was Penney. Mom said that was too long and shortened my name to Peny. One day, much later in my life when I was learning more about myself, I went to a psychic who told me that my middle name, Wilberta, meant healer. The name had been given to me in honor of my paternal grandfather, Wilber, who had been a wolf hunter and died before I was born. As for the rest, never would I nor anyone in my family or community ever have imagined I would have the experiences that would lead to so many last names.

My little girl self had been free and safe with a strong, although unconscious, sense of being. I got much of that from my paternal grandmother Cleo, whom I called Amo, and also from the land we lived on. Our ranch connected to the Black Hills National Forest and looked down the valley into South Dakota from Wyoming.

One afternoon when I was about four, Amo and I walked up the canyon that was just behind our house. "Peny," she said, "come let me sit you on the branch of this tree." Laughing with delight, I rode this imaginery box elder tree horse while my grandmother picked thimbleberries nearby. I tumbled onto the grass and lay there. I was part of the woman picking berries, I was the berry. I knew this, just lying there feeling the earth with my body. I never shared this feeling with my family. I didn't believe they would understand.

As an adult woman, I heard people speaking in amazement about out-of-body experiences. My own amazement stemmed from the realization that I'd been doing that since I was a child. I'd be lying in bed, waiting to fall asleep, when suddenly I'd be in a corner of the room, hovering at ceiling height, watching myself sleep. Then I'd be out in the night, playing among the stars. I never experienced my return, I'd just be back in my body when I woke in the morning.

The same with my dreams. They were, and are, vivid and very real to me. I was four years old the first time I had my vampire dream. I awoke, terrified, got out of bed and crawled in with Amo, snuggling up to her warmth and trying to recover from my fear. I couldn't possibly have known that this dream would recur every time I went through major life changes.

Even though I knew my family loved me and took good care of my physical body, I felt I couldn't trust them with something else about me, something I didn't understand, though I could feel it.

One day, when I was about seven, the morning sun warmed me as it poured through the open door of the cabin my great uncle Homer had built on our ranch. He was a mountain man who had lived with the Indians and had come to our ranch an old man. After suffering a stroke, my family placed him in a nursing home. Later, Dad let my brother and me have the cabin for "our house."

I had been sweeping the wooden floor in my bare feet when warmth from the wood moved from my soles up through my whole body. I stood quite still in what seemed to me to be a pool of joy. Bzzz, bzzz. A fly buzzed lazily in the corner of the window. Behind me the cast-iron wood cookstove stood silent, as if glad of my presence but sad that its warming ovens and reservoir were not in use. The heavy workbench, with its foot-thick plank top and handmade wooden vise, sat just under the north window where the light came in brightest for fine work.

To the west sat Uncle Homer's bed, its metal frame softened by the handmade patchwork quilt, heavy for warmth and lined with a wool blanket. An old rocker faced the potbelly stove just behind the cookstove, for warmth between meals. His taxidermy tools lay in the corner. Under the south window was an old grub box Uncle Homer had used for storage—three feet by five feet and heavy-built to last for the overland passage. He'd saved it out of the wagon that had brought our kin west in 1879. Table, cupboard, cabinet and washstand filled the rest of the space in this place that had been his home.

Way back, at the base of my tongue, I tasted the freshness of the air, like clear water from our spring located up the canyon. I smelled cinnamon, and ginger, and remembered Uncle Homer's fresh biscuits covered with wild plum butter, made of plums picked from the bush outside his door.

A gentle breeze rustled the leaves on the plum bush. Oak brush tapped at the window. A meadowlark joined in the chorus, and once more the fly went bzzz, bzzz.

Down the valley shadows played tag over the red butte, as small clouds raced to become thunderheads.

I was suddenly aware, for the first time, of myself as a separate, complete being. I stood feeling my being, and also my connection to this land, in a powerful way that would last all my life. Bzzz, bzzz. Lazy fly, or maybe just contented, like I was.

This feeling of being connected lasted until I was nine, when I joined 4-H and began to belong to the community instead of to myself. My actions no longer affected only me.

The year I was eleven I took sewing as one of my 4-H projects. "Peny," Mom said, "we're going to town to pick the fabric." I chose coral and turquoise with dancing girls for the skirt and plain coral for the blouse and apron. Both my mom and grandmother checked on me frequently and gave me encouragement as I learned to sew a straight seam. Our treadle sewing machine allowed me to go slowly. It was important that I get it right. At last I finished and the time had come for the county style review. That was when the girls who had taken sewing gathered to be judged by Home Economists, on our finished garments and how we presented them.

At the far end of the stage, I paused. Excitement wrestled with fear as I swallowed the lump in my throat. I heard the narrator say, *"Peny Goodson,* modeling her skirt, blouse and apron." Those words were my cue. I walked slowly to center stage, paused, turned and untied my apron. After carefully laying it over my arm, I turned and smiled at the judge. I had a smile that lit up the room. Slowly I walked off the stage and down the stairs. I'd won a purple ribbon, the grand championship of my division.

One night when I was about thirteen, my family and I went to a 4-H achievement celebration. I had gone out to a car with other boys and girls and we were all giggling and having a great time. Suddenly, my dad yanked open the door and grabbed my arm. Pulling me from the car he shouted, "Peny, how can I ever trust you again?"

Sex hadn't even entered my mind, but my father seemed to believe I was deliberately doing something to shame him and his good name in the community.

My family made it clear to me, without it ever being stated, that I was to do the best, be the best, and never do anything that didn't bring credit to the Goodson name.

One day, during my freshman year of high school, one of the "older men," a junior, approached me. "You're such a snob, Peny Goodson. Always having your nose in the air, I'm surprised you don't drown." I was devastated and ran sobbing to the girls' bathroom. My girl friends gathered around me, assuring me that he was dumb and not to worry, who was he anyway? My heart raced and my stomach felt queasy. As I cried I thought to myself, what else could he think? My folks wouldn't let me date, my grades were better than his, and every time I joined an organization I worked hard to become its president. *Penelope Perfect*, that was me. I wondered if I would ever smile again.

I did smile again. That boy was the first one who ever kissed me.

During this time my horse was my best friend. With him there were no expectations, all I had to do was ride.

Dad had brought him home, one evening, from the livestock sale he'd gone to that day. The horse was a three-year-old sorrel quarter horse with a white blaze in the middle of his forehead. He'd been abused so was head shy, but Dad figured he'd get over that with my loving attention. I named him Red because of his color.

We lived eleven miles from Sundance, Wyoming. At fifteen I was able to get a driver's license, and from then on drove myself and my brother to town for school. Dad wanted us home right afterwards for supper regardless of what was going on in the evening—meetings, ball games or play practice.

"Hurry up," I'd call to my brother, "I want to get home in time to ride before it gets dark." My record for the eleven-mile drive from town to our ranch, in the days before our road was graveled, was nine minutes and forty-five seconds. I sped along, driving as I always did, looking forward to seeing Red. My brother swears to this day that his nerves of steel are a direct consequence of those rides home from school.

Running up the walk I see steam on the kitchen window. Opening the door I am met by the warm smells of Mom and Amo canning corn. "Corn for supper?" I ask as I run to change my clothes. On my way back out Mom says, "Everything for supper's from the garden." Ymmm, I think, as I go to get a bucket of oats.

"Here Red, here boy," I call as I shake the bucket. He whinnies as he races to greet me. Whoa boy, you'll get your oats after our ride. Steady now, let me fasten your bridle.

He nuzzles me, impatiently wanting to be off and running. I buckle the chin strap and crawl on bareback. Feeling the warmth of his body through my legs, I lean over and give him a hug.

I urge him away from the gate with my knees, softly talking with him as I ride. "How was your day, boy," I say, as I proceed to tell him of mine. We've gone far into the lower pasture when I realize it is getting dark. "Time to go home," I say to him, as we turn toward the house.

I feel his muscles shudder in anticipation of our race home. I lean low over his neck, grasp his mane, let out the reins and whisper, "Run, boy, run." He stretches out his neck and runs, flat out like the wind. I laugh with pleasure as we skim the prairie grass. Eyes watering and hair flying we make for home. Coming to the last quarter mile before the gate I gently pull on the reins and say, "Easy now boy, whoa, we're almost there."

He stops, sides heaving. "You've earned your oats, boy," I say, as I slip from his back and undo the bridle. "Good boy," I say, as I hug him while he eats the oats. "See you tomorrow."

Most of my energy was devoted to my studies and organizations. I won nearly every award 4-H could present and if I hadn't gotten married when I was in college, would have been an International Farm Youth Exchange (IFYE) person , the highest honor bestowed by 4-H. I was also an officer in Future Homemakers of America, Future Teachers of America, Girls Athletic Association and the Episcopal Youth Club.

I was twenty-one when I married for the first time. That year I also got pregnant and graduated from college. Nothing—not 4-H, not school, not my family or doing well at nearly everything I did—prepared me for the next fifteen years of my life. I call it my roller coaster ride. It included three husbands, two children, two college degrees, fifteen moves, seven jobs (once fired), perfect homemaker, milk-and-cookies mom, 4-H leader, Boy Scout den mother, Sunday school teacher, and finally, the rebel I'd missed being when I was a teenager.

Fifteen years of a roller coaster ride seemed enough. I'd moved to Wyoming from Colorado with my third husband and believed my life was in order. I was pleased to be back in my home state. My kids were adjusting well to the move and I was thinking that our life looked like *House Beautiful*. We'd just moved to our new home when I celebrated my thirty-sixth birthday. That night I dreamed about my vampire, the dream I'd first had when I was four years old. I'd dreamed the vampire when my brother was born, when I began my menstrual cycle, went away to college, was divorced the first time and just before I was widowed. I woke up the next morning feeling anxious and as I lay there, realized I suspected my husband was having an affair with his secretary.

Two months later they ran away together. I'd treated him like a god, this young man who I believed had saved me from my grief, and this was my payback. I'd never allowed my feelings to surface when I was divorced the first time or when I was widowed. Both times I had my children to support and believed painful feelings were luxuries I couldn't afford.

The day the sheriff delivered divorce papers to my house, all this pent-up grief, pain and rage burst out of me. I lost thirty pounds in thirty days. I was in trouble and needed help. I'd asked my priest, one of the first women ordained to the priesthood by the Episcopal church, to be my counselor. One day, during my session, she said, "Peny, go have your vampire dream analyzed. You're dying before my eyes and I don't know what else to do for you."

I was fortunate that a woman trained in Jungian psychotherapy was practicing in Laramie. I called and made an appointment.

When I entered the room, I felt immediately at ease. The therapist was soft, round and beautiful. The picture of a goddess I'd been reading about came into my mind.

"Peny," she said, "the way I work a dream is to have you tell it to me. Then I'll write down your associations and we'll look at the meaning together. What's most important about Jungian dream analysis is that it is your process. What your unconscious reveals to you is all important."

I was relieved to hear that I'd be engaged in this experience and excited to be learning about my unconscious. Having received a graduate degree in psychology, I'd been to many therapists and often felt as though we were just exchanging psychobabble. I hoped that learning from my dreams would be different, because I was worn out from grief and needed something in my life to change.

"Now, you can tell me a dream that you want to know about," she said. I related to her my vampire dream.

"I'm a young woman, dancing with a dark handsome man. I wear a long, full ball gown. The ballroom is heavily draped in velvet. As we dance, the room begins to grow smaller and smaller. I look up at my partner and see that he is a vampire. Terrified, I wake up."

She wrote as I spoke. When I had finished, she said, "Peny, I want you to tell me the first association that comes to your mind when I mention these words. Please don't edit, just tell me the very first thought that comes to mind."

I breathed deeply and prepared to answer. The first words she said were "young woman."

"Me," I answered. She went on to ask about words from the rest of the dream and I supplied answers: dancing, fun; dark handsome man, energy; long gown, elegant; heavily draped velvet, elegant; smaller and smaller, suffocating; vampire, bloodsucker and taker of life.

After I'd finished giving her my associations, the therapist explained that my dream was giving me information that would help me take better care of myself. The questions she then asked helped me to understand what she meant.

What was I doing to suffocate myself? How was I sucking my own blood? Because, she told me, everything in the dream had to do with me and not with someone else! Could I see how these two things might be keeping me from a life of fun, energy, and elegance? In looking at those questions and considering my answers to them, I began to see a part of myself I'd never seen before—my unconscious.

For years I'd believed that my dad or my husbands were causing me pain. I'd never had anyone before who helped me to lovingly look at myself. Laying blame on others had been easier, but it hadn't worked. No wonder I was stuck in my grief.

I left my first session feeling I'd been given a breath of fresh air. For the first time in a long while I experienced a sense of hopefulness. No more psychobabble, but real information from my unconscious that would help me to heal. A few days later, on my way to work, I burst into song. I was so startled I nearly drove off the road. Me singing? I hardly dared to believe it. I was exhilarated and alive!

I continued having my dreams analyzed. Glen Carlson, a Jungian Analyst from Denver, became my analyst and mentor. Few things I'd ever done before had been so interesting. I had tapped into an unending source of information that was going to help me to truly become acquainted with my "self."

Learning about my dreams and integrating my unconscious were most important to my having had the courage to choose loving myself to health after my cancer diagnosis. If I'd never learned about my vampire, I'm sure that the bloodsucking, debilitating energy that he symbolically represents would have directed me toward turning my life over to the doctors instead of accepting personal responsibility, and seeking alternatives for healing.

After my biopsy, I had watched as the doctor marked X's all over a chart showing the outline of a woman's body. "Peny," he said, "do you have any cosmetic reasons for not having your breasts removed?"

He went on to say that he would need my permission to do anything he believed was necessary once he began surgery. "I'll remove the lump," he said, "but if I see that more needs to be done, I want to be able to do what I believe is best." In other words he wanted me to sign a release giving him permission to remove both breasts and all of the glands in my upper torso if he believed it was necessary. No more discussion or consideration. I was looking at the possibility of coming out of surgery totally mutilated.

I stared at the chart. X's on both breasts and on most of the lymph glands. "This has nothing to do with cosmetics," I tried to say. The words never left my mouth.

If I hadn't learned from my unconscious how to love myself, I believe the intense fear I experienced listening to and watching the doctor mark those X's would have propelled me into the operating room. Once Norman got me out of the doctor's office, I began to breathe slowly, allowing myself to get hold of the fear so I could work with it and not let it consume me.

Fight, battle and struggle are all words associated with traditional cancer treatment. Working with my dreams, I'd learned a long time ago that fighting never accomplishes anything. If my dreams hadn't told me, looking at the environment and the rest of the world would have. I chose to love myself to health. Except for the biopsy, nothing I've done has been invasive or painful. I've experienced no side effects and have felt good every day. In choosing love, I've chosen life. My focus is on how to live each day. I do not fear death. To me death is not the enemy. Not being healthy is my enemy.

I've paid attention to what I've been thinking as well as what I've been doing. I am conscious, thanks to my dream work.

Jacob Needleman, a philosopher who has written many books, including *Consciousness and Tradition* (Crossroad Publishing, 1982), says we need to be mindful. To be mindful is to be conscious and pay attention.

At a lecture I attended in 1972 in Denver, Victor Frankl, holocaust survivor and author of *Man's Search for Meaning* (Pocket Books, 1959), said that what Americans need is a Statue of Responsibility on the west coast to balance the Statue of Liberty on the east coast.

The woman I am today, loving myself to health and deepening my spiritual connection to all life, exists because I have become conscious and accepted responsibility for my life. In doing these things I have been given the gift of freedom to learn from all that is the worst in me and to become all that is the best.

Most importantly I have never lost, despite whatever has happened, the sense of belonging that the land at the ranch has always given me.

One winter day, in November of 1992, I climbed to the red cliff above and northeast of Uncle Homer's cabin. Behind me was a sentinel pine that had survived the fire of 1936. I sat looking at the cabin, scanning the valley, inhaling the chill air with its scent of oak and pine. It was so quiet that I felt as though I had dropped back in time one hundred years ago, and was alone in the universe.

Energy surged through my body from the earth. Around me, in the pine trees, chipmunks and squirrels raced from branch to branch as below me wild turkeys pecked for seeds. Nearby, a coyote spoke as I watched an eagle glide down the face of the mountain.

A lump formed in my throat. I felt the way I had on that long ago day when I'd stood barefoot in the cabin. All these things, I realized, were manifestations of the mystery of life I called The Creator. The love and connection I felt here filled me.

Pffft, Pffft. The sound was so soft I nearly missed it. I blinked to clear my sight and looked carefully around me. Snow was falling. I was hearing snowflakes light beside me. Pffft. Filled with wonder, I sat there knowing myself to be blessed, and once again knew of my being, separate but forever connected.

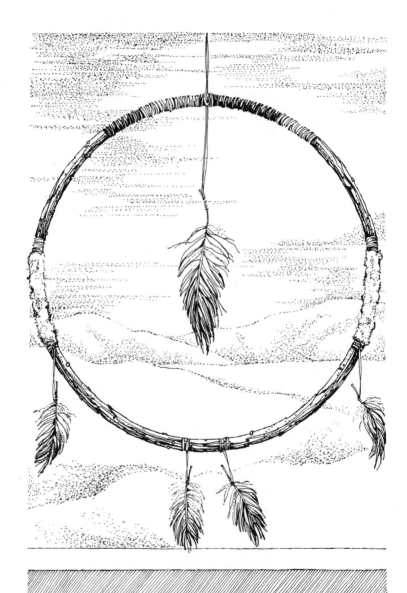

CHAPTER FIVE

Spirit

My experiences with spirits and their guidance

Not only was I connected to the land, I was connected to the spirits. About a week after my diagnosis, the spirit energy of my friend who had died two weeks before came to me. I'd been sitting quietly, meditating.

"Peny, Peny," a voice called. Startled, I looked up. To my right, about two feet away, was the image of my friend.

"Hi," I said, and smiled. It was wonderful to see him, looking like his old self. The last time I'd seen him he was skin over bone.

"Peny," he said, "I've come to give you support for the choice you've made about healing your cancer. I'll be right here, whenever you need encouragement." As he spoke he raised his right fist in a gesture of power. That's how he appeared to me each day after that, urging me on with my healing. At night, the vision changed. I'd see him running with a herd of buffalo. His vitality and joy were obvious. I'd go to sleep feeling totally at peace. His spirit energy stayed with me for several months. One day, he spoke again.

"Hi Pen," he said. "I see you're firmly on your way to making the changes necessary to be healthy. I'm going now. If I'm needed, let me know and I'll be back."

"Thanks," I said. Thanks felt inadequate, but I knew he understood exactly what I meant. I felt comforted and encouraged by his support. He comes back, now and then, just checking in when I'm feeling completely alone. He was a good friend to me and his spirit energy has continued to be a blessing.

I'd grown up terrified of death. One of my earliest memories is of my grandmother and father grieving my grandfather's death. Something about their grief felt inconsolable and I hated that. When I'd see pictures of death or someone in a parade portraying The Grim Reaper, wearing a black hooded cape and holding a scythe, I was sure he would get me. At night, if I were out by myself, I'd be afraid that a skeleton hand might grasp me from behind and pull me into the underworld. It wasn't until my second husband was killed, and I had firsthand experience with death, that I saw there was no reason for fear. Just after his motorcycle accident, he was taken to the hospital.

When I arrived I saw that his boots were pointing straight up, not relaxed, and I knew he was dead. His eyes were open and his pupils were steel grey. He was lying there, on the hospital bed, with a beautiful, peaceful expression on his face. I realized that he was no longer in his body and that he was happy wherever he had gone. It came to me that my fear of death had been fear of the pain that comes with grieving.

When I was diagnosed with breast cancer, I knew how lucky I was not to be afraid of dying. My nutritionist had told me she'd seen women die from their fear, not from the illness.

Early on, as I brought together as much information and support as possible, I called my mentor, Glen Carlson, who had been my analyst for a number of years. A few days after our conversation he sent me *Quantum Healing* (Bantam Books, 1989), a book by Deepak Chopra, M.D. Doctor Chopra is a practicing endocrinologist, former chief of staff of New England Memorial Hospital in Stoneham, Massachusetts, and founding president of the American Association of Ayurvedic Medicine. In the note that was enclosed, Glen commented that Marian Woodman, a Jungian Analyst from Toronto, Canada, whom I had met and respected, had recommended *Quantum Healing* as an excellent resource for me.

For many years I had tried to meditate but was frustrated because I couldn't clear my mind. Dr. Chopra says that meditation is nonjudgmental awareness of the self, not tuning out, but tuning in, being restful and alert. That's what I wanted, nonjudgmental awareness. I began practicing every day. The deep breathing I'd learned from my yoga teacher helped me to tune in to myself.

One morning I decided that while I was meditating I'd go inward to my memory of Uncle Homer's cabin. I wanted to try and contact the spirits of my ancestors, particularly my two grandmothers, Amo and Geomy. In my mind I went to the door of the cabin and sat down on the steps. Cougar, bear, snake, eagle, raven, horse, and mouse, creatures that support and comfort me as I meditate, were all with me. I told them I wanted to invite the spirits to come and help me. "All you have to do is ask," they said.

"How simple," I thought to myself. "But then most things of great value are."

They all came: my great-grandparents, grandparents and Uncle Homer. I looked at them sitting at the table in the cabin, and was filled with thankfulness. I'd been a little afraid they'd ask me to join them but chose to take the risk.

We sat together in silence for a while. Then I said, "I need your help. I want to be well and healthy. Can you send energy to me as I heal?"

In unison, they all nodded. They talked among themselves for a while and then Geomy said that she and Amo would stay with me, in spirit, while everyone else sent energy. They agreed that I got good feelings from Uncle Homer's cabin and encouraged me to continue with my meditation.

I thanked them all with love, hugged my cougar and ended my morning meditation.

I'm a person who likes to touch things, so I decided to wear Amo and Geomy's rings.

"Mom," I said, when she answered the phone, "I wonder if I could borrow Geomy's red ring? You know, the one with silver filigree that has a pear-shaped red stone. I've been meditating, and Geomy and Amo's spirit energies are going to help me. I want something that I can touch whenever I need to be reminded they're with me. I already have Amo's wedding ring and I want Geomy's ring to wear with it."

"I don't want to send it in the mail, but you can get it the next time you come up," Mom said.

"Thanks, I'll talk with you again soon. Love you," I said, and hung up the phone.

I'd become very particular about who I talked to on the phone, so I always enjoyed my mom. I'd stopped talking with people who were sending me their fear. Cody, a young friend with whom I'd done dream work, helped me with the negative energy. I'd called his mom and asked if she'd have Cody call me when he could. He was away learning about aboriginal survival skills. When he got my message he asked his American Indian teacher to do a sun dance for me. I was honored when he called and told me a sun dance had been danced on my behalf. As we talked, he said he heard something in my voice that was unclear.

"It's the concern. It feels like anvils dropping on me and wearing me out," I said.

"Hang in there, Pen," Cody said. "I have an idea. You'll be getting a package in about a week."

"Thanks," I said. The love that was coming to me, from so many sources, filled my heart with warmth.

Sure thing, in a little over a week the mailman left a package. I opened the box and saw rose quartz and a warrior hoop. Rose quartz, Cody said in his note, was to help keep my heart open. The hoop was a ten inch circle made of willow. Red, green, gold and blue threads were wrapped at the top and on the sides. Feathers hung from the top, middle, sides and bottom. The hoop, Cody wrote, would help protect me from negative energy. It was golden eagle, raven, bending like the willow, colors of courage, strength, earth, and ass kickin'! That's Cody, honest and to the point. Tears of thankfulness slid silently down my cheeks as I hung the warrior hoop in my kitchen window, where it hangs to this day.

I was pleased, a few months later, to be able to thank Cody in person. I was traveling to visit my son in Arizona, and stopped at Cody's home. We were sitting, meditating together, when he exclaimed, "Peny, I thought you'd turned purple!"

I burst into laughter. "I'm wearing purple," I said. He grinned and told me he'd been holding me in purple healing energy, looked up and thought I'd turned purple.

I could easily have looked purple. A color for healing, it's one of my favorites and comforts me.

Cody gave me four large natural crystals to take home, to provide powerful energy for my continued healing.

When I meditate, both my grandmothers come to me in spirit. I wore their rings for months, but quit one day when my parents were visiting.

"Peny," asked my mother, "did you have your rings on when you scrubbed the toilet?"

"Yes," I replied, "I wear them all the time."

"Oh no!" she cried. "You'll ruin them!"

I was sure that Amo and Geomy had worn their rings while they did their cleaning, but I wasn't going to argue.

I wear the rings once in a while, because they're beautiful and bring joy to my heart, but I no longer need them as a reminder that my grandmothers' loving energy is with me.

During one of my meditations I was blessed with seeing beautiful energy particles that looked like gold dust, coming from the universe to help with my healing. The particles were gold, blue, purple and silver. The energy dust moved through me, cleansing and strengthening. I believe it held all of the love from people I love, as well as love from the universe.

After I saw this healing energy, I was fortunate to see energy, in colors of the rainbow, coming to the planet to heal all humans. When I spoke to someone about this, they said, "Then why, if humans are healing, are there so many catastrophes?"

For thousands of years, I believe, we've experienced a deep wounding of the soul. When any wound begins to heal, it hurts like hell. If the scab is knocked off, the pain becomes intense, but that's a sign it's getting well. This is how I feel about my own health. Sometimes my breasts hurt, but I know them to be healing. I am healing from the inside. Nasty stuff that has been in me for years is being pushed to the surface where it is expelled. I hurt sometimes, just as we humans experience the pain of pestilence, war, famine and natural disasters.

Something about the human condition reflects always being in a hurry. We want everything fixed yesterday even though it may have taken many years for the problem to occur. I've said for years I've needed a sign in my office that says, "Am I Done Yet?" This is sometimes how I feel about my returning to health, even though I know better. I believe the healing of all humans is the same.

Each time I've seen a baby born who is well loved, like my granddaughter, Paige, my belief about health is reinforced.

The loving spirit of my friend, my ancestors' spirit energy, the love of family and friends and the beautiful energy coming in from the universe are blessings for which I will always be thankful.

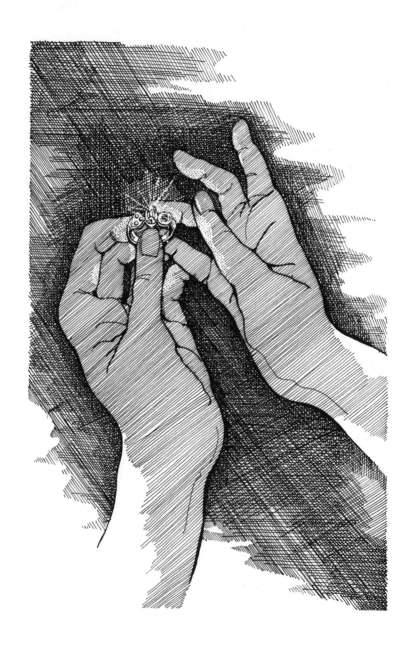

CHAPTER SIX

Diamonds Are Forever

Only when you buy them yourself

In *Jitterbug Perfume* (Bantam Books, 1984), Tom Robbins uses the term "Erleichda," lighten up. In choosing to be responsible for my life, I've also chosen to lighten up and to do more things for myself that are fun. Like my snake. I never imagined I'd get so hooked on its symbology that I'd have a ring, custom made, in the shape of a snake and wear it every day. I'm a person who likes to see and touch symbols, not just talk about them.

I have a friend who is a jeweler. One day I walked into his store with the simplest sort of sketch and said, "I need you to make a snake ring for me."

He put down the pipe stone he'd been carving and said, "Let me see your idea."

I wanted the band to have the curved and graceful body of a snake, its head and tail meeting on each side of a healing ruby I'd been given at a women's vision quest. The body needed to be gold with tiny diamonds marking the head. I brought the ruby with me so that if he thought he could make the ring, he could begin right away.

"Sure thing," he said, "it will be ready in about two weeks. I'll call you."

I gave him a big hug and danced my way out his door. I was excited to be getting the ring.

When I'd begun to have my dreams analyzed, I realized how often I dreamed about snake. My analyst told me that, in the collective unconscious, snake meant healing and knowledge as opposed to the Christian consciousness that calls snake evil. The medical professionals have honored snake in their use of the caduceus, a symbol modeled on Hermes' winged staff with two serpents twined around it. I had come to believe that every time I dreamed snake my unconscious was trying to bring knowledge to me that would help me heal some pain I was or had been experiencing.

I had my first encounter with snake when I was five. A beautiful bull snake was entwined around the horseradish plant just in front of our woodshed. "Marjorie," my grandmother yelled to my mother, "come help me kill this snake."

Mom ran out of the kitchen and grabbed a short-handled shovel that stood in the corner of the shed.

Snake, who surely was wondering about all the commotion, began to uncoil and slide away.

"You pin him down, Marjorie, and I'll see if I can chop off his head."

Mom just caught his tail with the shovel, at which point snake reversed his course and began coming toward my mother. He was a long snake and that shovel handle was short. Mom backed up, farther and farther, yelling to my grandmother to cut off his head before he got to her. My grandmother succeeded.

I felt the greatest sadness. "Mama," I asked, "why did you have to kill the snake? Daddy says bull snakes keep rattlers away and he wasn't hurting anything."

"I won't have snakes in the yard," she snapped. My grandmother picked up snake's body and head and carried them out to the tall grass outside the back gate.

The next incident with snake occurred after a movie one evening when I was a teenager. We'd just turned onto the dirt road that led to our house when Dad yelled "rattlesnake" and brought the car to a sliding, dusty halt. He jumped out, got the tire iron out of the trunk and attacked the snake. Snake had coiled in defense of itself, and was striking. I had no thought for my Dad. A tremendous sense of desolation welled up from the pit of my stomach. Flashes of heat chased themselves over my breast, into my throat, behind my eyes and then down my arms. Tears blinded me as I began a scream that felt as if it would never stop. Dad killed the snake while my mother tried to comfort me.

To this day my parents have no idea I was grieving for the snake and not frightened for Dad.

Don't misunderstand me, if snake were to come sliding in through the door I would not walk over and calmly greet it. I'd be scared, I've been too well conditioned not to. I would, however, encourage it back outside.

One summer, not long ago, I ran out my back door and nearly stepped on a water snake that had been sunning at the bottom of the steps. My scream pierced the morning quiet, and my husband came running to see what was happening. "I just scared a snake to death," I said. I'm sure that was true. Anyone will strike when frightened, and I'm sure the snakes are as frightened of us as we are of them. When we pay attention to where we're going, we don't get into their space and have nothing to fear.

When I got my cancer diagnosis, my friend Linda said, "You know you're mortal now, Peny, don't put things off that are important to you."

I'd wanted a diamond ring for a long time. At a seminar Sam Keen, author of *The Passionate Life* (Harper & Row, 1983) and *Fire in the Belly* (Bantam Books, 1991), asked us to write titles for chapters of our lives. The first thought that came into my mind was "Diamonds are forever but only when you buy them yourself." I knew I wanted to buy my own diamond rather than have Norman get it for me as tradition suggests.

I went back to the jeweler and asked if he could find me a good quality diamond to fit my snake ring in place of the ruby. "I only have two thousand dollars," I said, "but this is really important to me."

He grinned, hugged me, and said he'd see what he could do. A few days later he called to tell me there might be a diamond that would work. The stone was in Denver and he needed my ring to check the size.

Later in the week I was walking across the street near his store when a sharp whistle caught my attention. "Pen, come see what I have for you," he yelled from his doorway.

I ran, pleasure flooding my body as though I were greeting a lover. The ring lay there in his palm with all the beauty I could ever have hoped for. I slid it onto my middle finger, trusting it was as glad to be there as I was to have it back. We smiled at one another as I walked around his store.

"You're acting just like a newly engaged woman," he said.

"I am. I've just become engaged to myself. What I've learned about being well is that I need to love myself. This ring, with snake and diamond, is to remind me that when I love myself and am open to the knowledge all around me, I am healing."

"What a great idea," he said.

Now, most times when he sees me he says, "So how are you and snake?"

"Healing," I reply, and smile.

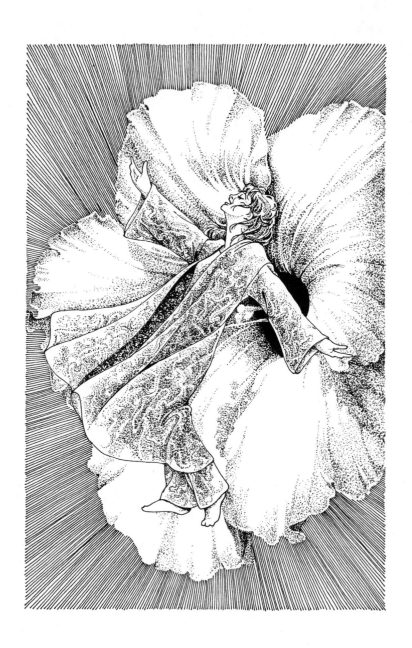

CHAPTER SEVEN

Nature's Wisdom

Naturopathy
and Homeopathy

After I had begun to learn about living in a healthy way, I had the good fortune to take a six-week trip to New Zealand and Australia. My husband had business in New Zealand, flying scientific balloons. His boss had given him time off, when the flights were completed, to travel with me. I relaxed, totally releasing myself to playtime with my husband.

Norman T. Kjome, my fourth husband, is the man who courted me for five years as we both healed from emotional wounds. We chose to marry because we trusted each other and had a wonderful passion between us.

I considered my cancer as a wake-up call to become healthy. We discussed what I was doing and what other things I wanted in my healing process. One thing we both agreed was important was for me to try to find a doctor who would support me in my natural healing.

A little over a year later, I prepared carefully for my meeting with the new doctor in town. He was a naturopathic and homeopathic doctor. He called his practice "In Nature's Wisdom." Until a couple of weeks before, I would have gone trustingly in to meet him. No more. I'd been laboring under the illusion that all alternative healing people were open and honest. I'd learned differently.

Two friends, on the same day, had given me the name and telephone number of a new acupuncturist with excellent credentials. When I called him, we had a good talk and I eagerly made my first appointment.

I should have suspected something the day I arrived at his office, because as I waited at the front door my car began to drive away. I flung off my sandals and raced barefoot after its slow moving form, thankful I hadn't locked the door. Running alongside, I caught the door handle, pulled open the door and got in, put on the brake and sat there shaking. Slowly I started the car, backed up and parked, this time remembering the emergency brake.

I walked back to the house to wait. The acupuncturist had told me he'd be late. Soon a car drove up and a young man got out and came toward me. I was still unsettled by my car incident, so I just smiled, held out my hand and introduced myself. He took my hand and told me he was glad to meet me.

We entered his office. It was cold and sterile. The acupuncturist excused himself and returned wearing a doctor's smock. I knew he was very well trained and had hospital experience, but I hadn't expected such a clinical atmosphere. I was interviewed and given my treatment but I was not comfortable. The many questions I'd prepared went unasked. I had gone to other acupuncturists, all of whom had been warm and comforting. The difference I was experiencing did not make me happy.

I didn't have to make the decision whether or not to continue work with this person. He called me at home to tell me that because I had been diagnosed with cancer, and wasn't under the supervision of a medical doctor, he wouldn't work with me. I was shocked. I felt as if he had found something that suggested my impending death and instead of telling me the truth was choosing not to work with me. I realize this sounds irrational. That's how I felt. It took me days of concentrated work to recover from what seemed like another body blow. I would never again trust anyone who called themselves healer until I had personal experience of them.

Getting ready to see Michael Lang, the naturopath and homeopath, I put on my power clothes, the outfit I wear when I know I don't want anyone to mess with me. It's purple, blue, orange and black. It flows around me and I feel vibrant, just like the colors. Next I wrote out two questions on a 3x5 index card. 1) Are you afraid of cancer? 2) Do you believe in spiritual healing? I was ready.

Dr. Lang greeted me and asked if I'd like some tea. As we settled into our chairs I began, "I realize I'm here to learn something of what you do, but first I have a couple of questions I want to ask you." He looked slightly startled but smiled and said, "Sure." I asked my questions. To my great relief he wasn't afraid of cancer and, he believed in spiritual healing.

I relaxed, took a sip of my tea, and studied this man as he began to tell me about his way of healing.

Dr. Lang was tall, slender and easy with himself. His hands were long and looked to be both capable and gentle. A beard. I was pleased. I'm partial to men who wear beards, no doubt because I have such a passion for my husband and he's worn one since I've known him. Graying, dark brown hair, fine facial features and warm, hazel eyes. Dr. Lang looked like a strong, passionate man and felt like a breath of fresh air.

His idea of responsibility, both his and mine, toward my continuing health was what I'd been seeking. I sighed and felt tears well in my eyes. At last, someone knowledgeable who would support me in my healing. We made a deal: I wasn't there about cancer and he wasn't treating me for cancer. I signed the agreement. What a treasure this man was, trained in medicine but understanding immediately that my issue was bringing my life into balance and loving all of me, not fighting cancer.

"Michael," I said, "I want you to know I prayed you up." He smiled and didn't seem to mind. I think he was as pleased to have someone who was willing to work toward health as I was to have found him.

I began a program called P.E.P., the Personalized Education Program. The purpose of P.E.P. is to promote exceptional health, one step at a time. I had already begun. For over a year I'd been working hard detoxing. I supported my cleansed system with nutritious food, supplements, yoga and walking, as well as quiet time to relieve stress and make contact with my spiritual being.

Homeopathy is a way of healing that involves taking minute doses of various natural substances which interact with your biochemical nervous system, causing whatever has been promoting disease in your system to move out.

During the fourteen years I had been involved in Jungian psychoanalysis, my task had been to peel the onion from the outside in, removing the layers of information that had separated me from myself, to get to my essence.

Homeopathy did the reverse, beginning with the core of the onion, the source of dis-ease, pushing out layer by layer until the stressors that had been working, emotionally and physically, for dis-ease were cleaned out and the self was free and clear.

Michael listened carefully to everything I said to him during several consultations. He gave me a thorough physical exam, and two series of chemical workups from my blood.

When all the information had been carefully analyzed, Michael gave me a remedy that would work with my issue of world pain. For many years I had felt what seemed to be all of the pain of the world. Coupled with the many intense personal experiences I'd had, which I'd referred to as my roller coaster ride, it didn't take a rocket scientist, as my brother would say, to find a central reason for my body's imbalance. Michael told me that as the remedy worked I'd probably feel more emotion and anger than usual. I hadn't looked forward to that experience but I believed it would be worth added intensity in my life to move the world pain out. This was in the fall, so I had Thanksgiving and Christmas, holidays involving many expectations for me, which added fuel to the fire of my intensity. I was not sure I'd survive Christmas. My emotions were stirring and cooking like a huge cauldron and I didn't feel well.

Nevertheless, I survived. At the end of December my husband went to the Arctic for his yearly research trip. I was left with a lot of personal time and space. I put an electric mattress pad on the bed so I'd be warm and well rested.

One morning in early January, I awoke to the light. I lay in my bed quietly, with my eyes closed, as intense feelings filled me. I felt myself to be light. My breath came from the bottom of my lungs, gusting upward as the pain of the world dropped from me. I saw, in my mind's eye, myself leaving the planet as though I were a space shuttle. Pieces of me named violence, injustice, betrayal and pollution, no longer needed for my flight, were falling off, burning in the atmosphere below. I had lived my life believing all these things to be my responsibility and that I was to right all wrongs.

I didn't move but lay there breathing deeply, air continuing to gust from my lungs. A sharp pain, between my breasts, caught at my breath. The pain broke, like a bubble bursting. I was free from my burden of world pain. Sleek and powerful, I winged my way toward continued healing.

Michael had told me he was from Montana and loved it there. One day, about nine months after we'd begun our work together, he said, "I'm moving my family to Kalispell." Both of us had tears in our eyes at the thought of him going.

"I know this is the right thing for you to do Michael," I said, "because you'll be licensed in Montana and I know that's important, but"—I took a deep breath as I tried to steady my voice—"what am I going to do without you?" I wanted to throw my arms around his legs and hang on, wailing my sense of loss.

He took my hand and I sat there, crying quietly. One of the wonderful things about Michael was that he was a fully present person. When I was with him I always knew his energy was totally focused, there with me.

I withdrew my hand, blew my nose and said, "So what am I going to do?"

"I will always be available by phone, Pen," he said, "but there is another possibility. A woman I went to school with is opening a practice in Colorado. I think you met her at the Mountain Healing Center. I'd like you to call her. If you feel comfortable with her, I'll send your records and she will be your doctor.

I smiled, knowing he wanted the very best for me. I realized that he was having mixed feelings, was glad to be getting back to Montana but sad to be leaving his patients. I hugged Michael when I left, promising to make an appointment with Anne Scott, the doctor he'd recommended.

I was always pleased when I'd meet healers who were sure enough of themselves to allow patients to call them by their first names. Michael and Anne both preferred first names to Dr. Lang and Dr. Scott.

I made an appointment with Anne a couple of months after Michael had moved. I'd called him a few times, but both of us agreed I needed someone I could speak with face to face, and someone I could hug. We knew we'd stay in contact, but I needed a doctor closer to home.

I found Anne's office easily, and went in to her waiting room.

"Hi," she said. "You must be Peny. I'm Anne Scott. Come on back to my office."

We smiled at one another and I followed her. The office, flooded with sunshine, had many plants and a rocking chair for me to sit on.

"I'm going to do a review so I'll feel up-to-date with what's happening with your health. Michael sent me your records so we won't have to do a complete intake. I already have a lot of information."

I felt relaxed and comfortable, sitting in the rocker.

"It looks like you're taking many supplements," she said.

"Yes," I responded, "and I feel like I'm about to overdose. I want to continue to be healthy but this is just too much."

"Come into my examining room and I'll do muscle testing with you so we can see which ones you can quit taking."

I'd brought all of my supplements in a bag so I picked it up and we went to the next room.

"Hold your right arm straight out. When I press down try to hold it firm." She took each supplement, one at a time, and held the container with a magnet to my stomach as she pressed down on my arm. Each supplement that I no longer needed caused my arm to stay firm. My arm would drop when she held those I still needed.

The magnet inverted the usual reaction to muscle testing. When my arm stayed firm, it meant that the supplement was not good for me or was neutral. When my arm dropped, it meant that the supplement was good for me.

When we'd finished, I saw that I only needed about three-fourths of what I had been taking. This now included my herbal compound, a multivitamin, some digestive enzymes, vitamin E, a complex of nutritional and herbal support tablets, concentrated salmon oil, calcium and magnesium, beta carotene, milk thistle combination and vitamin C.

"That's better," Anne said. "We'll keep working so that you have even fewer things to take, but for right now this looks good."

After the muscle testing, she examined the lump in my breast. As my body was healing the last couple of years, the mutated cells had been contained in the one lump. There were no tumors anywhere else in my breasts or my glands.

Anne was an attractive, slender woman with brown hair and green eyes. From the moment I'd entered her space I'd been at ease.

We returned to her office and the rocking chair.

"Peny," she said, "I want to try a homeopathic remedy that I think may shrink your tumor."

"Sounds good to me," I said.

"Check in with me in a couple of weeks and let me know how you're feeling."

"Bye," I said, "and thanks." We hugged and that ended my first visit.

I've continued to see Anne every six weeks or so. We've worked with my becoming menopausal and continued work with my immune system which has become healthy. I've had blood work done verifying its recovery.

My tumor is shrinking. I rub it every night with a healing oil, phytolacca, and thank it for my many lessons. My tumor has kept me honest, reminding me to always love my body.

I was forty-nine when I found the cancerous tumor. Since then, healing my body has been an adventure.

Dr. Chopra says that the whole body rejuvenates in seven years. I can think of nothing more worthy than being fifty-six with a new body. What a great way to begin the second half of my life.

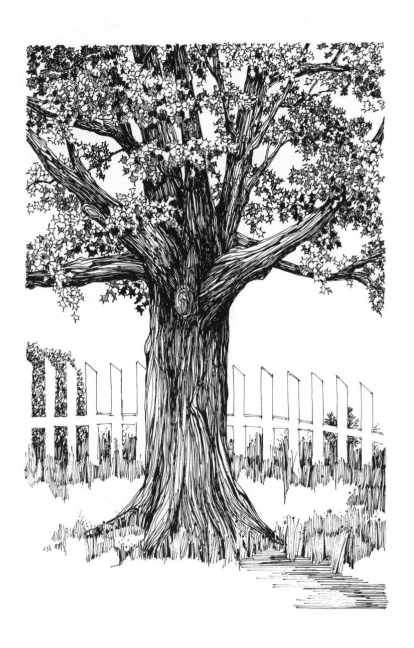

CHAPTER EIGHT

Being Human

Finding balance and
the lessons I have learned

I still have dark days. I get tired and would rather be perfect instead of human. Forget balance. I want someone else to be responsible for me. Why should I have to work this hard? It's not fair. Nothing is okay, I'm never going to get anything I want. No one can help me, fix it or make it go away. Everything is hopeless. That's a dark day.

If only I could shut off the voice in my head that speaks to me when I've been too busy to take time for myself.

"Peny, you must be stupid or crazy. Of course you should have had surgery, at least a lumpectomy. How can you possibly imagine that you are healing without doing what the doctor told you to do?"

I drop into depression, feel totally alone, weep, scream and swear. In the midst of this tirade another voice is heard.

"What are you doing? Be still and count your blessings."

That voice reminds me of what my analyst had said to me.

"Peny, until you learn to count your blessings, nothing will really work for you. I can't believe that if you give up what you perceive as your responsibility for the world that you'll begin throwing beer cans out of your car windows."

How right he was. Once I breathe deeply and become quiet, it's simple for me to count my blessings. And, I haven't thrown anything out of my car windows.

I had been told to keep my sense of humor since I was still human. The Creator had said that if I chose to live, there would still be pain, violence, injustice and pollution in the world. I didn't want to believe it. I wanted to stay in my body but I didn't really want to be human, experiencing all of life including pain and despair.

The first time I felt depressed, after I had been learning how to take care of myself, I was disappointed. I had been sure that every day of my life I'd be so glad to be alive I'd never be depressed again.

Not true.

As I breathed deeply and began to move out of the depression, I looked at what was happening, trying to find the reason. That's when it came to me: this is what balance is about—good and bad days. The American Heritage Dictionary, Third Edition, says that balance is "a stable state characterized by cancellation of all forces by equal opposing forces." In this culture we've been so busy pursuing happiness I believe we've lost sight of what it means to be in balance. By choosing to pursue health, instead of happiness, I hope to come into balance.

I had begun my healing reading *Walk In Balance*, by Sun Bear, and then lost sight of what I'd learned, that I'll experience joy and pain, love and anger. I will not always be in a state of bliss. I change just like everything else in life. I am alive, not static. I ebb and flow just like the sea. When I am in balance I am healthy and powerful.

When I am out of balance I take my blessings for granted and become self-righteous. I begin to behave as though I know all the answers and can fix everyone if only they'd listen to me. I believe I'm being loving when I'm really being judgmental. This is particularly true with my family. One evening the phone rang.

"Hi Mom," said my daughter.

"Hi, sweetheart, you sound awfully tired," I said. "I wish you'd take better care of yourself. I'm sure you know better than to wear yourself out like this. I'll be angry if you make yourself sick."

"Gee, Mom," she said, "I just called to see how you are, not to get a lecture."

"I'm sorry, Jamie, I know you take good care of yourself. What's going on that you're so tired?" I asked.

She went on to tell me about her day and I realized she really did know how to take care of herself. I needed to remember that. When I am unloving to others I am also unloving to myself. Then it's depression and the dark days are with me. I am, however, beginning to appreciate those times, knowing they will never feel good but are necessary for my balance.

I believe it's important to write down the lessons learned from any life experience, especially dark days. When I am clear about the lesson, then hopefully I will move on to new lessons without having to repeat the old ones over and over again. I never want to be diagnosed with cancer again, so what lessons have I learned? I want to share the most important ones.

Fear often appears to be in control of the world, especially in the Western medical establishment. It's fight this and battle that. I chose not to live in fear. I am loving myself to health.

When I look at my fear I see I do have choices. In fear, there is no choice.

I am living, not surviving.

My body is as important to me as my spirit, psyche, emotions and intellect.

I live in integrity with myself, speaking my truth.

Being Human

There is nothing more important to me than my life.

Everything that lives has as much right on the planet as I do. I have more responsibility because I am human.

Understanding is not necessary for love, but acceptance is.

Doing is not always best. Often it does more harm than good. Being is something I'd like to allow.

I have a right to my opinion. I also have the responsibility to be clear that it is only my opinion, not the law nor the word of God.

I make mistakes, that's how I learn. Forgiving myself for making mistakes is important so that I can learn from them. It also allows me to forgive others so that they, too, can have the freedom to learn.

I must love myself before I can love others.

The only way I can listen is to be quiet.

The most important time in my life is now. The past is finished, the future unknown.

"Judge not lest ye be judged" is true. How I treat others is how I am treated.

Change is necessary for life.

Life and death are part of the whole, two faces of the same coin.

I need growing things in order to be healthy.

Everyone has a path. No one's path is exactly the same. I respect that truth.

Money is not evil. Money made from fear, however, I see as evil.

My life is my own and I am one with The Creator.

Concern feels heavy to me, not loving.

All information has value.

I am loved and I love.

Quality of life is more important to me than quantity.

I no longer know for others, only for myself.

It is not only acceptable, it is necessary that I say no, in order to be healthy.

In order to be healthy, I must count my blessings and be thankful.

Becoming aware of these lessons meant that as I moved through my initiation toward becoming a healer, I was learning to walk in balance.

There is no ending to my story. I continue to be healthy, to learn and to count my blessings.

Appendix, Reading List and Index

Appendix

This outline for healthy eating is only a guide. You will discover what makes your body feel its best and then make your own outline.

I have included recipes for bran muffins and two soups which helped sustain me as I sorted out what worked the best for me. In the beginning, they were especially satisfying and I have not grown tired of them. The soups keep well, so they can be made in larger amounts and eaten over several days. After you start looking, you will be able to find many wholesome recipes in various vegetarian cookbooks.

Outline for Healthy Eating

BREAKFAST
Fresh fruit
Granola (low fat, low sodium), with unsweetened
  fruit juice

10:00 AM
Bran muffin with nuts and fruit
Fresh fruit

LUNCH
Organic or kosher poultry, fish, cage-free eggs
Mixed vegetable juice (low sodium)
Whole grain bread, crackers
Brown rice, buckwheat, beans
Soup
Salad (low-fat dressing)

3:00 to 4:00 PM
Mixed vegetable juice (low sodium)
Fruit
Bran muffin
Juice from juicer (e.g., carrot, celery)

SUPPER
Pasta with meatless sauce
Beans
Vegetables
Rice, buckwheat, quinoa, couscous
Soup (no meat)
Whole grain, seed bread, crackers
Salad (no meats or cheese)
Stir fry, oriental foods (no MSG)
Liquid aminos for seasoning

BEDTIME SNACK
Fresh fruits (good time for citrus—orange,
 grapefruit)
Herbal tea
Vegetable juice

ALL DAY
Chamomile, raspberry leaf and other herbal teas

SNACKS
Raw almonds, sunflower, pumpkin seeds (no salt)
Popcorn, no butter, a bit of salt or liquid aminos
Raisins, dates, currants
Almond butter, molasses, maple syrup

NO POULTRY, FISH, EGGS after 2:00 PM
USE VERY LITTLE SALT, SUGAR, or FAT
NO DAIRY, PORK, LAMB, BEEF
NO FRIED FOODS (except stir-fry)
NO SAUCES, CHOCOLATE, COFFEE, TEA (except
  herbal teas)
NO SOFT or DIET DRINKS (except natural drinks)
REMEMBER TO EXERCISE
Walking, yoga and jumping on a mini-trampoline
are excellent!

RECIPES

Bran Muffins
1 cup bran
2 cups bran cereal
1 cup boiling water

Mix ingredients and let stand a few minutes.
Add:
1/2 cup oil (canola)

2 eggs or 3 egg whites or 1/2 cup Eggbeaters
2 1/2 cups whole wheat flour
2 1/2 teaspoons baking soda
1/2 to 3/4 cup oatmeal
2 cups orange juice
Mix and add dates, nuts or raisins as desired.
Spices may be added.
Bake at 375 degrees for 20 minutes.

Pea and Lentil Soup
12 cups of water
1 small onion
2 carrots
4 stalks of celery
2 potatoes
Chop all vegetables

1 cup green split peas
1/2 cup lentils
1/2 cup adzuki beans
2 teaspoons olive oil
1 bay leaf
1 teaspoon basil
1 teaspoon thyme
2 tablespoons of vegetable boullion or broth mix
Put all ingredients in a large pot with a lid. Bring to
a boil. Turn heat down and simmer for 2 to 2½ hours.
Makes 10 cups.

Kashi ® Soup

2/3 cup lentils

2/3 cup split peas

2/3 cup Kashi, uncooked

1 garlic clove, peeled and minced

1 small onion, chopped

1 stalk celery, chopped

1 carrot, peeled and chopped

8 cups vegetable broth

1 teaspoon paprika

1 teaspoon salt

1/2 teaspoon black pepper

pinch of dried thyme

Wash the lentils, split peas, and Kashi in cold running water and drain. Put them in a 4-quart saucepan.

Add all other ingredients to the saucepan and cook, covered, over moderately low heat for 1 hour, stirring occasionally, or until lentils, split peas and Kashi are soft. Serves 6.

Kashi ®, Seven Whole Grains and Sesame, is a registered trademark of Kashi Company, La Jolla, CA. Used with permission. Kashi Pilaf can be found in grocery, specialty and natural food stores.

Reading List

Health

Bach, Edward, and F.J. Wheeler. *The Bach Flower Remedies*. New Canaan, CT: Keats Publishing, Inc., 1979.

Bertherat, Therese, and Carol Bernstein. *The Body Has Its Reasons: Self-Awareness Through Conscious Movement*. Rochester, VT: Healing Arts Press, 1989.

Brown, Raymond Keith. *AIDS, Cancer and the Medical Establishment*. New York: Robert Speller Publishers, 1986.

Carter, Albert Earl. *The Cancer Answer*. Scottsdale, AZ: A.L.M. Publishers, 1988.

Chopra, Deepak. *Quantum Healing*. New York: Bantam Books, 1989.

Diamond, Harvey and Marilyn. *Fit For Life*. New York: Warner Books, Inc., 1985.

Frazier, Barbara. *The Wholefoods Menu Book*. Huntington Station, NY: Lifestyle Series Publishers, 1983.

Gerson, Max. *The Cancer Therapy*. Bonita, CA: Gerson Institute, 1958.

Griscom, Chris. *The Ageless Body*. Galisteo, NM: Light Institute Press, 1992.

Hanna, Thomas. *Somatics: Reawakening the Mind's Control of Movement, Flexibility, and Health*. Reading, MA: Addison-Wesley Publishing Co. Inc., 1988.

Haught, S.J. *Has Dr. Max Gerson A True Cancer Cure?* North Hollywood, CA: London Press, 1962.

Hay, Louise L. *You Can Heal Your Life*. Santa Monica, CA: Hay House, 1984.

Heimlich, Jane. *What Your Doctor Won't Tell You*. New York: Harper Perennial, 1990.

Jackson, Mildred, and Terri Teague. *The Handbook of Alternatives to Chemical Medicine*. Oakland, CA: Lawton-Teague Publications, 1985.

James, Walene. *Immunization: The Reality Behind the Myth*. South Hadley, MA: Bergin and Garvey Publishers, Inc., 1988.

Kabat-Zinn, Jon. *Full Catastrophe Living: Using the Wisdom of Your Body and Mind to Face Stress, Pain and Illness*. New York: Dell Publishing, 1990.

Kelly, William Donald. *One Answer to Cancer*. Grapevine, TX: Kelly Research Foundation, 1967.

Kervran, C. Louis. Translation and Adaptation by Michel Abehsera. *Biological Transmutations*. Magelia, CA: Happiness Press, 1978.

Louden, Jennifer. *The Woman's Comfort Book*. New York: Harper San Francisco, 1992.

Moss, Susan. *Keep Your Breasts!: Preventing Breast Cancer the Natural Way*. Los Angeles: Source Publications, 1992.

Parvati, Jeannine. *Hygieia, A Woman's Herbal*. Berkeley, CA: Bookpeople, A Freestone Collective Book, 1978.

Percival, Mark. *Functional Dietetics, The Core of Health Integration*. New Hanburg, Ontario, Canada: New Health Perspectives Inc., 1991.

Reilly, Dr. Harold J., and Ruth Hagy Brod. *The Edgar Cayce Handbook for Health Through Drugless Therapy*. New York: Jove Publications, 1975.

Weed, Susun S. *Menopausal Years: The Wise Woman Way*. Woodstock, NY: Ash Tree Publishing, 1992.

Whitmont, Edward C. *Psyche and Substance: Essays on Homeopathy in the Light of Jungian Psychology*. Berkley, CA: North Atlantic Books, 1980.

Worsley, J.R. *Acupuncture, Is it for You?*. Longmead, Shaftesbury, Dorset, Great Britain: Element Books Limited, 1988.

Wright, Jonathan V. *Dr. Wright's Book of Nutritional Therapy.* Emmaus, PA: Rodale Press, 1979.

Psychology

Frankl, Victor. *Man's Search for Meaning.* New York: Simon and Schuster, 1959.

Gawain, Shakti. *Creative Visualization.* New York: Bantam Books, 1983.

Hannah, Barbara. *Encounters with the Soul: Active Imagination as Developed by C.G. Jung.* Boston: Sigo Press, 1981.

Harding, M. Esther. *Woman's Mysteries: Ancient and Modern.* New York: Harper and Row, 1971.

Johnson, Robert A. *She: Understanding Feminine Psychology.* New York: Harper and Row, revised edition, 1989.

Johnson, Robert A. *He: Understanding Masculine Psychology.* New York: Harper and Row, revised edition, 1989.

Jung, Carl G. *Memories, Dreams, Reflections.* Recorded and edited by Aniela Jaffé, Translated from German by Richard and Clara Winston. New York: Vintage Books, 1965.

Mindell, Arnold. *Working with the Dreaming Body.* Boston: Routledge and Kegan Paul, 1985.

Peck, M. Scott. *The Road Less Traveled*. New York: A Touchstone Book, Simon and Schuster, Inc., 1978.

Pincolas Estes, Clarissa. *Women Who Run with the Wolves*. New York: Ballantine Books, 1992.

Robbins, Anthony. *Awaken the Giant Within*. New York: Simon and Schuster, 1991.

Shinoda Bolen, Jean. *The Tao of Psychology: Synchronicity and the Self*. Toronto, Canada: Inner City Books, 1982.

Philosophy

Keen, Sam. *Fire in the Belly*. New York: Bantam Books, 1991.

Keen, Sam. *The Passionate Life*. New York: Harper and Row, 1983.

Keen, Sam. *Hymns to an Unknown God: Awakening the Spirit in Everyday Life*. New York: Bantam Books, 1994.

Needleman, Jacob. *Consciousness and Tradition*. New York: Crossroad Publishing, 1982.

Sacred

Blum, Ralph. *The Book of Runes*. New York: St. Martin's Press, 1982.

Campbell, Joseph. *Myths To Live By*. New York: Bantam Books, 1973.

Chief Archie Fire Lame Deer and Helene Sarkis. *The Lakota Sweat Lodge Cards: Spiritual Teachings of the Sioux*. Rochester, VT: Destiny Books, 1994.

Gibran, Kahlil. *The Prophet*. New York: Alfred A. Knopf, Publisher, 1967.

Moore, Thomas. *Care of the Soul: A Guide for Cultivating Depth and Sacredness in Everyday Life*. New York: Harper Collins Publishers, 1992.

Summer Rain, Mary. *Earthway: A Native American Visonary's Path to Total Mind, Body and Spiritual Health*. New York: Pocket Books, 1990.

Sams, Jamie, and David Carson. *Medicine Cards: The Discovery of Power Through the Ways of Animals*. Santa Fe, NM: Bear and Company, 1988.

Sun Bear, Crysalix Mulligan, Peter Nufer and Wabun. *Walk in Balance*. New York: Prentice Hall Press, 1989.

Zurkav, Gary. *The Seat of the Soul*. New York: Simon and Schuster, 1990.

Other

Robbins, Tom. *Jitterbug Perfume*. New York: Bantam Books, 1984.

Index

Index

Personalized Education Program 93
Prayer 33, 46
Protein 43

R
Radiation 9-10, 21, 28
Recipes 111-113
Red meat 47
Reflexology 51
Relaxed 89
Relaxing 31
Runes 52

S
Salt 45, 47
Sense of humor 48
Shaving 47
Snacks 111
Snake 27, 29, 76, 84-87
Soups 32, 112-113
Spirit 73-74, 76, 104
Spirituality 31
Spleen 50
Steam baths 45
Stress 53
Sugar 49
Sun Bear 31-32, 102
Supplements 48
Support 73
Symbols 83

T
Teague, Terri 32
The Creator 19, 22, 32, 35-36, 53, 102, 106
Toxins 30, 36, 43, 46, 50

Notes